SpringerBriefs in Education

We are delighted to announce SpringerBriefs in Education, an innovative product type that combines elements of both journals and books. Briefs present concise summaries of cutting-edge research and practical applications in education. Featuring compact volumes of 50 to 125 pages, the SpringerBriefs in Education allow authors to present their ideas and readers to absorb them with a minimal time investment. Briefs are published as part of Springer's eBook Collection. In addition, Briefs are available for individual print and electronic purchase.

SpringerBriefs in Education cover a broad range of educational fields such as: Science Education, Higher Education, Educational Psychology, Assessment & Evaluation, Language Education, Mathematics Education, Educational Technology, Medical Education and Educational Policy.

SpringerBriefs typically offer an outlet for:

- An introduction to a (sub)field in education summarizing and giving an overview of theories, issues, core concepts and/or key literature in a particular field
- A timely report of state-of-the art analytical techniques and instruments in the field of educational research
- A presentation of core educational concepts
- An overview of a testing and evaluation method
- A snapshot of a hot or emerging topic or policy change
- An in-depth case study
- A literature review
- A report/review study of a survey
- An elaborated thesis

Both solicited and unsolicited manuscripts are considered for publication in the SpringerBriefs in Education series. Potential authors are warmly invited to complete and submit the Briefs Author Proposal form. All projects will be submitted to editorial review by editorial advisors.

SpringerBriefs are characterized by expedited production schedules with the aim for publication 8 to 12 weeks after acceptance and fast, global electronic dissemination through our online platform SpringerLink. The standard concise author contracts guarantee that:

- an individual ISBN is assigned to each manuscript
- each manuscript is copyrighted in the name of the author
- the author retains the right to post the pre-publication version on his/her website or that of his/her institution

Thanat Tangpaisarn · Paul E. Phrampus ·
John M. O'Donnell

Navigating Healthcare Simulation

A Practical Guide for Effective Teaching

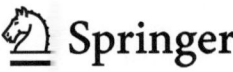 Springer

Thanat Tangpaisarn
Emergency Department
Faculty of Medicine
Khon Kaen University
Khon Kaen, Thailand

Paul E. Phrampus
Winter Institute for Simulation, Education,
and Research (WISER)
University of Pittsburgh
Pittsburgh, PA, USA

John M. O'Donnell
School of Nursing
Winter Institute for Simulation, Education,
and Research (WISER)
University of Pittsburgh
Pittsburgh, PA, USA

ISSN 2211-1921   ISSN 2211-193X (electronic)
SpringerBriefs in Education
ISBN 978-3-031-81264-4   ISBN 978-3-031-81265-1 (eBook)
https://doi.org/10.1007/978-3-031-81265-1

This Springer imprint is published by the registered company Springer Nature Switzerland AG
The registered company address is: Gewerbestrasse 11, 6330 Cham, Switzerland

If disposing of this product, please recycle the paper.

Simulation is a technique—not a technology—to replace or amplify real experiences with guided experiences.

—David M. Gaba

Preface

This book is crafted for both novice simulation educators embarking on their teaching careers and seasoned subject matter experts seeking to enhance the effectiveness of their simulation programs. The book draws on the effort of a novice simulation educator under the guidance of two simulation experts with over 40 years of collective experience.

Embark on a transformative journey with our book, *Navigating Healthcare Simulation: A Practical Guide for Effective Teaching* is designed to empower readers who utilize simulation as a teaching tool. This book serves as a roadmap, leading educators toward a more organized and practical approach to conducting simulations.

Covering a wide spectrum of topics, the book begins with insights into associated learning theories for simulation, providing valuable strategies for increasing learner engagement. Delving deeper, it explores various simulation modalities and locations, guiding educators to choose the best options for their teaching objectives.

Within the pages of this handbook, readers will find detailed discussions on scenario design, simulation phases, and the crucial aspect of debriefing. In addition, the book addresses learner assessment and course evaluation, ensuring a well-rounded understanding of the entire simulation process.

We invite our readers to explore the wealth of knowledge within these pages, with the hope that you will gain valuable insights to elevate your simulation skills and contribute to the continuous improvement of your teaching practices.

Khon Kaen, Thailand
Pittsburgh, USA
Pittsburgh, USA

Thanat Tangpaisarn
Paul E. Phrampus
John M. O'Donnell

Contents

Chapter 1
Introduction to Healthcare Simulation

Abstract This chapter provides a comprehensive historical overview of healthcare simulation, tracing its origins from ancient China to the aviation industry's influence in the early 1900s. Pivotal moments in medical simulation evolution, including the development of wax anatomical models and Resusci Annie and SIM one mannequins, are highlighted. Moving to the contemporary landscape, the chapter defines healthcare simulation as a methodology for practice, learning, and system evaluation, emphasizing its role in developing essential cognitive, technical, and behavioral skills for healthcare professionals. The multifaceted purposes of simulation, advantages such as improved patient safety, and limitations like cost and fidelity are explored. The chapter concludes by previewing subsequent sections that will delve into effective strategies for simulation-based education, underscoring its critical role in modern medical education and practice.

Keywords Medical simulation evolution · Cognitive skills development · Patient safety · Simulation-based education · Healthcare simulation evolution

1.1 History of Healthcare Simulation

Approximately a millennium ago, in 1027, during the Song Dynasty in China, the imperial physician Wang Wei-Yi employed life-sized bronze statues as a pedagogical tool for teaching the art of acupuncture (Owen, 2012). Additionally, wax body parts had been used as votive offerings in Catholic churches in Florence from the thirteenth century. Ludovico Cardi used this technology to produce the first wax anatomic model in the sixteenth century (Ballestriero, 2010). In the eighteenth century, in Bologna, Italy, Giovanni Antonio Galli, a surgeon by trade, conceptualized a birthing simulator. It was reported as a device featuring a glass uterus nestled within a pelvic structure, housing a fetus. This invention was intended to serve as a training aid for midwives and surgeons, facilitating the mastery of childbirth techniques. These examples offer a glimpse into the early roots of simulation in medical education.

T. Tangpaisarn et al., *Navigating Healthcare Simulation*,
SpringerBriefs in Education, https://doi.org/10.1007/978-3-031-81265-1_1

The rise of modern healthcare simulation can be linked to the aviation industry, which underwent a pivotal transformation in the early 1900s. A series of catastrophic airline accidents, often attributed to poor visibility, prompted a paradigm shift in pilot training. The adoption of simulation approaches was a significant advance and as these methods became more sophisticated, aviators were offered a safer, more cost-effective avenue to hone their skills, including during emergency situations (http://www.starksravings.com/linktrainer/linktrainer.htm; Rosen, 2008). World War II added momentum to the adoption of simulation technology, with military applications extending beyond aviation. Other high-risk sectors, such as submarine operations and space exploration, also embraced simulation for training. This period witnessed the genesis of simulation's journey from the skies to the broader spectrum of high-stakes industries (http://www.starksravings.com/linktrainer/linktrainer.htm).

The healthcare industry also learned and benefited from this promising approach. In nursing, the first mannequin used to teach nurses was a life-size doll know as Mrs. Chase. She was built in 1911 by Martha Jenkins Chase (a doll maker) for the Hartford Hospital (Hartford, CT) to train nurses to dress, turn, and transfer patients (Aebersold, 2016). In 1960, a seminal moment in medical simulation occurred with the invention of Resusci Annie, a simulation device manufactured by the Laerdal corporation. Based on the work of three individuals often referred to as the 'fathers' of CPR, Drs. Peter Safar, William Kouwenhoven, and James Jude, this device was initially conceived for mouth-to-mouth resuscitation training and marked a significant milestone in the history of simulation in healthcare education (Aebersold, 2016; Rosen, 2008) (Fig. 1.1). In 1966, the University of Southern California unveiled a rudimentary yet groundbreaking creation: a full-scale human patient anesthesia simulator named Sim One. It represented a collaboration of engineering, industry and medical expertise between engineer Stephen Abrahamson, physician Judson Denson, and Aerojet General Corporation. Sim One displayed lifelike facial features including blinking eyes, adjustable pupils, and an articulating jaw. Its chest region mimicked respiratory movements and synchronized heartbeat with carotid and temporal pulses, complete with a simulated blood pressure response. Moreover, the mannequin could emulate reactions to specific drugs and allow for basic airway management procedures (Abrahamson et al., 1969; Rosen, 2008).

Since these pioneering milestones, the utilization of simulation in healthcare has undergone a remarkable evolution, with applications across a wide array of clinical disciplines. Healthcare domains, including emergency medicine, surgery, critical care, anesthesiology, nursing, and pharmacy have embraced simulation as an invaluable tool for education and training, enhancing the competence and confidence of students as well as healthcare practitioners.

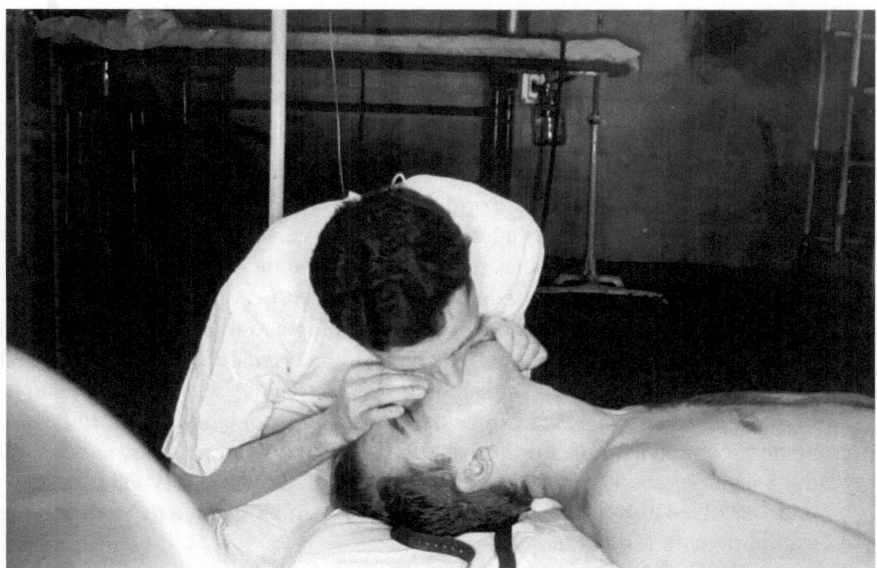

Fig. 1.1 Dr. Safar's early tests of his CPR technique on volunteers at Baltimore City Hospital (*source* Box 30 Folder 2, Peter Safar Papers, 1950–2003, UA.90.F102, University Archives, Archives & Special Collections, University of Pittsburgh Library System)

1.2 What Is Healthcare Simulation?

Healthcare Simulation, or Clinical Simulation, is a methodology using various modalities that create a situation or environment to allow persons to experience a representation of an actual healthcare event for practice, learning, or evaluation of systems and human actions. In modern healthcare education, simulation is an immersive experience used to educate healthcare professionals and support their development of key cognitive, technical, and behavioral skill sets that can be transferred to actual clinical practice. Through the use of simple to technologically advanced simulators, experiences can be designed to allow students as well as practicing healthcare professionals to gain the knowledge, skill and confidence (KSA) needed to develop competence without the fear of harming a patient or delaying the diagnosis and treatment of actual patients (https://www.ssih.org/About-SSH/About-Sim ulation Lopreiato 2018; Phrampus, 2023a).

1.3   Purposes of Healthcare Simulation

Healthcare simulation is a versatile methodology using a wide range of simulation devices and applications that can be used to address a number of academic domains (https://www.ssih.org/About-SSH/About-Simulation; Phrampus, 2023a), including:

- **Education**: Healthcare simulation provides a platform for the development of critical knowledge, skills, and attitudes (e.g., confidence, self-efficacy) that support the development of competencies needed to improve their abilities in delivering high quality patient care. This educational approach occurs in controlled environments designed to allow critical decision-making and to provide feedback on the quality and safety of care, thus safeguarding real patients from the potential risks of trainees gaining these skills in the clinical arena. A wide variety of simulation devices and approaches can be used, ranging from simple task trainers to computerized mannequins. Further, the use of standardized patients, augmented reality systems, screen-based simulations, and full virtual reality environments have also evolved as important approaches that can implemented to 'scaffold' the education process for learners.
- **Assessment**: Healthcare simulation plays a pivotal role in evaluating the competence of healthcare students, practitioners, and teams as well as environments of care. This dichotomy of assessment can be conceptualized as individual and team development versus probing of the environment or system for safety or process flaws. From an individual or team standpoint, assessment approaches range from low-stakes exercises aimed at improvement (formative assessment) to high-stakes assessment designed to gauge an individual or team's competency (summative assessment). When using simulation for an assessment of the practice environment or healthcare system, critical information such as latent patient safety threats, equipment presence and or placement, and other system factors can be assessed.
- **Research**: Healthcare simulation is a valuable tool for exploring individual/team competence, clinical protocols, risky procedures and new technologies. By simulating various scenarios and measuring outcomes, researchers seek to gain insight into how these performances, protocols, procedures, or technologies function. This information can then be used to identify areas for improvement as well as potential risks. The outcomes of simulation research are often divided into (1) improvement of the participant's/team's performance in the lab and clinical setting, (2) improvement of actual patient care, and (3) improvement of the actual patient care environment (McGaghie et al., 2011)
- **Systems Integration**: Healthcare simulation centers and educators are ideally positioned to design and implement approaches that can be used to facilitate the integration of simulation into institutional training and healthcare delivery systems. This integration has the potential to bolster patient safety and elevate the quality of care by offering a safe and effective training environment. Additionally, it aids in evaluating organizational processes, enhancing overall efficiency and effectiveness.

1.4   Advantages of Healthcare Simulation

Healthcare simulation offers a plethora of benefits, underscoring its pivotal role in modern medical education and practice (https://www.ssih.org/About-SSH/About-Simulation; Lateef, 2010):

- **Patient Safety**: Simulation provides a secure and controlled environment for students and healthcare professionals to practice various skills and procedures. This invaluable feature ensures that patients remain safeguarded from potential harm, reducing medical errors and elevating overall patient safety.
- **Assured Access to Key Experiences**: Traditional learning and skill acquisition often relies on learners' random encounters with relevant cases. This haphazard approach means that there is wide variability in student learning. In contrast, simulation offers the opportunity for targeted and focused learning experiences that are difficult to obtain in real life. These learning opportunities can be scheduled at convenient times and locations and repeated as often as necessary.
- **Tailored Learning Activities**: Simulation can be meticulously customized to align with the specific needs of individual learners or organizations. This adaptability allows for a highly personalized learning experience, ensuring the training directly applies to each learner's individual learning objectives and can be modified for a variety of work settings.
- **Evaluative Potential**: In real healthcare settings, the fast-paced nature of operations often leaves limited room for in-depth analysis and reflection on the care provided and analysis of the "why" and "how". Simulation, on the other hand can be designed to facilitate an assessment of healthcare professional skill, knowledge and attitude. Evaluation approaches can assume various forms, including through observation, focused testing, and post-simulation debriefing sessions. Through assessment, areas requiring improvement can be identified, enabling ongoing tracking of the learner's progress and growth.

1.5   Limitations of Healthcare Simulation

Healthcare simulation offers significant benefits for enhancing healthcare professionals' and students' competence and knowledge. However, like any tool, it comes with its own set of limitations (http://www.academyprodev.com/1/post/2017/01/pros-and-cons-of-simulation-in-healthcare.html; Phrampus, 2023b):

- **Cost**: The acquisition of simulation equipment can be financially daunting. These expenditures can pose challenges, particularly for institutions with limited resources. Further, the cost of sustainment can be even more challenging as the overhead for simulation centers, personnel and maintenance of devices can be a substantial ongoing cost.

- **Availability**: Simulation equipment may not be universally accessible across all healthcare settings. Some institutions may lack the resources or infrastructure to incorporate a broad range of simulation activities into their training programs.
- **Fidelity**: The degree of realism in simulation equipment can vary widely. Many simulators only partially replicate real-world scenarios, impacting the authenticity of the training experience.
- **Interpretation of Data**: The outcomes of simulation exercises can be complicated to interpret. Analyzing and drawing meaningful conclusions from data acquired during simulation activities may pose challenges due to the presence of a number of confounding variables. Approaches to reduce variability in data include use of highly structured and validated simulations, programming of simulation devices to enhance reliable patient presentation, and training of instructors and raters.
- **Translation to Clinical**: While simulation has proven invaluable for skill acquisition in the simulation lab setting, there is no guarantee that these skills will seamlessly translate to real-world clinical settings. Bridging the gap between simulation and actual practice can be challenging but is necessary for quantifying the value of this educational methodology.
- **Simulation Sickness**: A subset of individuals may encounter simulation sickness (AKA cybersickness), a phenomenon characterized by feelings of nausea, dizziness, and disorientation during the use of augmented reality (AR) and virtual reality (VR) simulation environments. This discomfort can hinder the effectiveness of the training and is usually limited to simulation encounters employing headsets. Attempts to modify this effect by reducing exposure time and allowing participants to gradually accommodate have demonstrated some success in the reduction of this limitation.

Subsequent chapters will explore strategies for successful, efficient, and effective design and implementation of simulation-based education. We will also provide strategies to mitigate some of the limitations discussed to optimize the benefits of healthcare simulation.

References

About Simulation. Accessed September 5, 2023. https://www.ssih.org/About-SSH/About-Simula tion

Abrahamson, S., Denson, J. S., & Wolf, R. M. (1969). Effectiveness of a simulator in training anesthesiology residents. *Journal of Medical Education, 44*(6), 515–519. https://doi.org/10.1097/00001888-196906000-00006

Aebersold, M. (2016). The history of simulation and its impact on the future. *AACN Advanced Critical Care, 27*(1), 56–61. https://doi.org/10.4037/aacnacc2016436

Ballestriero, R. (2010). Anatomical models and wax Venuses: Art masterpieces or scientific craft works? *Journal of Anatomy, 216*(2), 223–234. https://doi.org/10.1111/j.1469-7580.2009.01169.x

Lateef, F. (2010). Simulation-based learning: Just like the real thing. *Journal of Emergencies, Trauma, and Shock, 3*(4), 348–352. https://doi.org/10.4103/0974-2700.70743

Link trainer restoration. Accessed August 31, 2023. http://www.starksravings.com/linktrainer/lin ktrainer.htm

Lopreato, J. O. (2018, August 1). *How does health care simulation affect patient care?* Accessed September 1, 2023. https://psnet.ahrq.gov/perspective/how-does-health-care-simulation-affect-patient-care

McGaghie, W. C., Draycott, T. J., Dunn, W. F., Lopez, C. M., & Stefanidis, D. (2011). Evaluating the impact of simulation on translational patient outcomes. *Simulation in Healthcare, 6*(7), S42–S47. https://doi.org/10.1097/SIH.0b013e318222fde9

Owen, H. (2012). Early use of simulation in medical education. *Simulation in Healthcare, 7*(2), 102. https://doi.org/10.1097/SIH.0b013e3182415a91

Phrampus, P. E. (2023a, August 24). What is healthcare simulation? *Simulating Healthcare.* Accessed September 1, 2023. https://simulatinghealthcare.net/2023/08/24/what-is-simulation-the-question-that-caught-me-off-guard/

Phrampus, P. E. (2023b, April 25). When simulation is NOT the answer. *Simulating Healthcare.* Accessed September 5, 2023. https://simulatinghealthcare.net/2023/04/25/when-simulation-is-not-the-answer-own-it/

Pro's and cons of simulation in healthcare. The Academy of Professional Development. Accessed September 7, 2023. http://www.academyprodev.com/1/post/2017/01/pros-and-cons-of-simula tion-in-healthcare.html

Rosen, K. R. (2008). The history of medical simulation. *Journal of Critical Care, 23*(2), 157–166. https://doi.org/10.1016/j.jcrc.2007.12.004

Chapter 2
Learning Theory in Healthcare Simulation

Abstract This chapter delves into the critical role of learning theories in the realm of healthcare simulation, providing an in-depth exploration of five prominent theories: Knowles' Andragogy, Bloom's Taxonomy, Miller's Pyramid, Kolb's Cycle, and the Kirkpatrick Evaluation Model. The chapter concludes by emphasizing the significance of selecting the appropriate learning theory based on specific learning objectives and learner levels. It highlights how understanding and applying these theories empower educators to design tailored, effective, and efficient learning activities in healthcare simulation. The integration of diverse learning theories contributes to a comprehensive and strategic approach in the ever-evolving landscape of healthcare education.

Keywords Learning theories · Andragogy · Bloom's Taxonomy · Kolb's Cycle · Kirkpatrick Evaluation Model

Having a good understanding of key learning theories is highly beneficial when navigating the world of healthcare simulation. Many different learning theories can be applied to healthcare simulation. Some of the most common theories include Knowles' Andragogy, Bloom's Taxonomy, Miller's Pyramid, Kolb's Cycle, and Kirkpatrick's Evaluation Model.

2.1 Knowles' Andragogy

Malcolm Knowles' andragogy is a theory of adult learning that emphasizes the learner's self-direction, experience, and motivation. These assumptions are based on the belief that adults differ from children in their learning needs and preferences. Adults are thought to be more self-directed, have more life experience, and are more motivated to learn when the learning is relevant to their personal needs (Clapper, 2010; Knowles, 1980).

Knowles' theory has four main assumptions:

- **Self–directedness**: Adults are motivated to learn to solve problems or improve **their skills**. They are not as motivated to learn by external rewards or punishments.
- **Reservoir of Experience**: Adults come to the learning situation with **a wealth of experience** that can be used as a resource for learning.
- **Readiness to learn**: Adults are motivated to learn **when they need** knowledge or skill.
- **Orientation to learning**: Adults are more likely to learn when the learning is **relevant** to their personal and professional lives.

Knowles' theory has been applied to a wide range of adult learning approaches, including healthcare simulation. In healthcare simulation, Knowles' theory can be used to design learning activities that are more effective in meeting the needs of adult learners.

Here are some examples of how Knowles' theory can be applied to healthcare simulation:

- **Use of learner-centered learning**: Learner-centered learning is an approach to learning that focuses on the needs and interests of the learner. This approach can be used in healthcare simulation by allowing learners to choose the topics they want to learn about and the activities they want to participate in.
- **Active learning**: Active learning is an approach that involves the learner in the learning process. This approach can be used in healthcare simulation by allowing learners to practice skills, solve problems, and collaborate.
- **Reflection**: Learners can be asked to reflect on their personal experiences and how they apply to each scenario. Each learning activity can be designed to help learners **apply their experience** to new situations (in the simulation) and thus improve their skills.

Knowles' theory is a valuable tool for educators who are using healthcare simulation. By understanding this theory and how it can be applied, educators can design learning activities that are more effective for adult learners.

2.2 Bloom's Taxonomy

Bloom's Taxonomy is a taxonomy of **learning objectives** developed by Benjamin Bloom and his colleagues in 1956. In 2002, a revised version of Bloom's Taxonomy was published. It is a way of classifying learning objectives into six levels of complexity, from the simplest to the most complex (Krathwohl, 2002).

The six levels of revised Bloom's Taxonomy are (Fig. 2.1):

1. **Remember**: The learner remembers or recalls information.
2. **Understand**: The learner understands the information and can explain it in their own words.
3. **Apply**: The learner can apply knowledge to real-world situations.

Fig. 2.1 Revised Bloom's Taxonomy

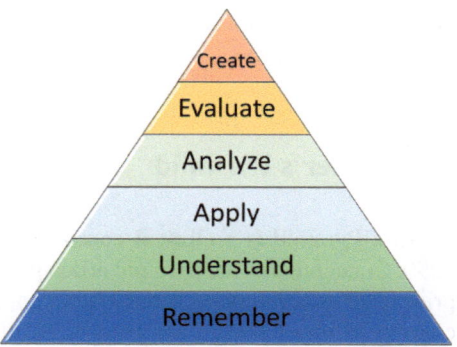

4. **Analyze**: The learner can analyze data acquired through learning and identify its components.
5. **Evaluate**: The learner can evaluate and judge the quality of the information being learned.
6. **Create**: The learner can synthesize data acquired through learning and create new ideas.

Bloom's Taxonomy can be used to design learning activities, assess learners' progress, and demonstrate the match of learning objectives to student level. As the student progresses from novice to expert performance, learning objective level should parallel student progression.

Here are some examples of learning objectives at each level of Bloom's Taxonomy:

- **Remember**: Learners are asked to recall the definition of asthma, recognize the symptoms of an asthma attack, and list the medications used to treat asthma.
- **Understand**: Learners are asked to explain the difference between asthma and other respiratory conditions, summarize the steps involved in an asthma action plan, and interpret the results of an asthma test.
- **Apply**: Learners are asked to identify the triggers for their patient's asthma, demonstrate how to use an inhaler, and apply the principles of asthma management to their own lives.
- **Analyze**: Learners are asked to differentiate between different levels of asthma, identify the causes of an asthma attack, and assess the effectiveness of different asthma treatments.
- **Evaluate**: Learners are asked to assess their own or other individuals' asthma knowledge and skills, and make judgments about the quality of asthma care.
- **Create**: Learners are asked to develop a plan for managing their patient's asthma, create a presentation about asthma, and design an educational intervention for people with asthma.

Bloom's Taxonomy is a valuable tool for simulation educators during both the design and assessment processes. By understanding the different levels of Bloom's

Taxonomy, educators can design learning activities that are more precisely aligned to learner objectives.

2.3 Miller's Pyramid

Miller's Pyramid is a **clinical competence** model developed by George Miller in 1990. Conceptually, the pyramid is designed to indicated that each level builds on the prior level as learners ascend. Concordant to Bloom's Taxonomy, Miller's Pyramid consists of four levels of competence (Miller, 1990) (Fig. 2.2).

1. **Knowledge (knows)**: The learner **knows** the facts and principles related to the clinical situation.
2. **Comprehension (knows how)**: The learner **understands** the facts and principles and can explain them to others.
3. **Application (shows or shows how)**: The learner can **apply** the facts and principles to real-world situations.
4. **Synthesis (does)**: The learner can **synthesize** the information from the clinical situation and develop a care plan.

As the learner is asked to demonstrate higher levels of competence, the requisite skill and knowledge required becomes more complex. Miller's Pyramid can be used to assess learners' progress and to design simulation learning activities that target specific levels of competence. For example, in a simulation, students may be required to retrieve specific knowledge facts (KNOW) and explain how the knowledge (e.g. medication dosage) should be applied during a simulation (KNOWS HOW). Then during the simulation the learner can be asked to administer the medication (SHOWS HOW). Ideally the learner would then have the opportunity to be observed actually administering the medication in a similar patient care situation (DOES).

Miller's Pyramid is a valuable tool for simulation educators in conceptualizing where elements of knowledge and skill can be applied and assessed. By understanding

Fig. 2.2 Miller's Pyramid

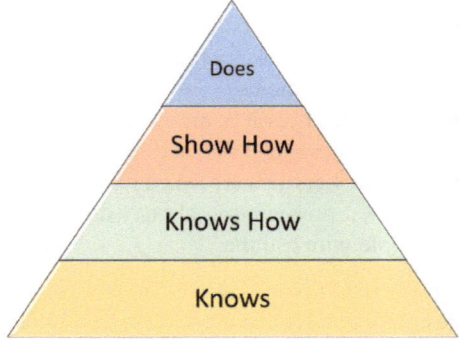

the four levels of competence, educators can design learning activities that support the learners' in meeting competency goals.

2.4 Kolb's Cycle

I hear, and I forget.

I see, and I remember.

I do, and I understand.

Confucius' quote summarizes Kolb's theory wonderfully, reflecting that a person learns in a number of domains but that action or doing is necessary for deeper learning.

Kolb views learning as a four-stage, continuous process where the participant acquires knowledge from each new experience. His theory treats learning as a holistic process where one continuously creates and implements ideas for improvement. According to Kolb, effective learning can occur when an individual completes a four-stage cycle (Kolb, 1984; Mcleod, 2022) (Fig. 2.3). The four stages of Kolb's Cycle are:

1. **Concrete Experience (feeling)**: The learner engages in an experience. This might be a new experience or situation, or a reinterpretation of existing knowledge in the light of new concepts.
2. **Reflective Observation (watching)**: The learner reflects on the experience and identifies what they learned.
3. **Abstract Conceptualization (thinking)**: The learner develops concepts and theories about what they learned.
4. **Active Experimentation (Doing)**: The learner then applies the concepts and theories to new situations.

Kolb's Cycle is a valuable tool for educators to understand that learning is not a linear process but involves a number of steps. By understanding the four stages of the cycle educators can design learning activities that support each step in the process. For example, in simulation scenario development, learners are asked to undergo a clinical-like experience. They are then debriefing and during the debriefing are led to reflect on their actions. At the end of the debriefing, the key points are summarized. These three steps reflect concrete experience, reflective observation, and abstract conceptualization. When they then engage in clinical practice and encounter a similar scenario, they have an opportunity to engage in active experimentation.

Following are some additional examples of how Kolb's Cycle can be used to understand how learners follow this process during healthcare education experiences in the clinical setting:

- A student is caring for a patient who is **experiencing** chest pain. The student engages in the concrete experience of interacting with the patient and assessing their condition.

Fig. 2.3 Kolb's Cycle

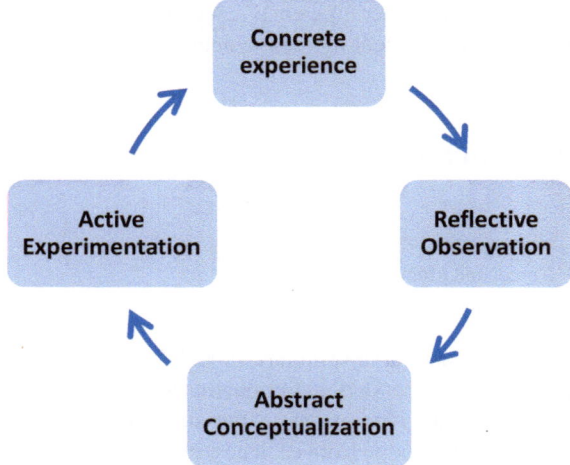

- The student then **reflects** on the experience and identifies what they learned, such as the patient's signs and symptoms, the appropriateness of interventions, and the importance of communication.
- The student then **develops concepts and theories** about what they learned, such as the pathophysiology of chest pain and the importance of teamwork.
- Finally, the student **applies** the concepts and theories to new situations, such as caring for a patient with a similar condition.

By understanding Kolb's Cycle, simulation educators can design learning activities that help students engage in the experiential learning process in the lab setting in order to develop the skills they need to be successful in the actual patient care environment.

2.5   Kirkpatrick Evaluation Model

The Kirkpatrick Evaluation Model is a four-level **framework for evaluating** the effectiveness of training and learning programs. Developed by Donald Kirkpatrick and James Kirkpatrick in 1959, this model has been widely used in various settings, including healthcare, business, and education (Kirkpatrick & Kirkpatrick, 2006).

The four levels of the Kirkpatrick Evaluation Model are:

1. **Reaction**: This level measures learners' **feelings** about the training program. Learners may be asked to rate their satisfaction with the program, the instructor, and the materials.

2. **Learning**: This level measures what learners have **learned** due to the training program. Learners may be asked to take a test or complete a performance assessment.
3. **Behavior**: This level measures how learners **apply** what they have learned in the training program to their work. Learners may be observed or asked to keep a journal of their progress.
4. **Results**: This level measures the training program's **impact** on the organization. This could include measures such as productivity, quality, or customer satisfaction.

The Kirkpatrick Evaluation Model can be used to evaluate the effectiveness of health care simulation in many ways. Some examples include:

- **Reaction**: Learners can be asked to **rate their satisfaction** with the simulation experience, the facilitator, and the course elements (e.g. equipment, supplies, simulators).
- **Learning**: Learners can be asked to **take a test** or complete a performance assessment to measure what they have learned due to the simulation experience.
- **Behavior**: Learners can **be observed** or asked to **keep a journal** of their progress to measure how they are able to apply what they have learned either in the simulation experience or in their clinical work.
- **Results**: The impact of the simulation experience on the organization can be measured by looking at measures such as **patient safety, quality, or cost savings**.

Here are some more specific examples of how the Kirkpatrick Evaluation Model can be used in healthcare simulation:

- A group of nurses are participating in a cardiac arrest simulation. After the simulation, the nurses are asked to **rate their satisfaction** with the experience and the facilitator. They are also asked to complete a **self-performance assessment** to measure what they have learned about cardiac arrest.
- After the simulation, the nurses are observed to see **how they apply** what they have learned during care of real-world patients.
- Finally, the hospital **tracks the survival rate or other patient-related outcomes** before and after the simulation training.

By using the Kirkpatrick Evaluation Model, healthcare organizations can ensure that their simulation programs are effective and meet their learners' and organizations' needs.

2.6 Summary

These are just a few learning theories that can be applied to healthcare simulation. The best theory for each planned simulation activity will depend on the specific learning objectives and the level of learners involved.

Once these factors have been considered, the educator can select the appropriate learning theory (ies) and design learning activities aligned with the theory. For example, if the learners are adult learners with prior experience in healthcare, then andragogy would be a good fit. The educator could design learning activities that allow learners to share their experiences, reflect on their practice, and apply their learning to new situations.

Kolb's cycle would be a good fit if the learning objectives were focused on clinical decision-making. The educator could design learning activities that allow learners to experience clinical scenarios, reflect on their decisions, and apply their learning to new scenarios.

If the learning objectives are focused on assessing learners' clinical competence, then Miller's pyramid would be a good fit. The educator could design learning activities that allow learners to demonstrate their knowledge, comprehension, application, analysis, and synthesis skills.

Learning theories can be a valuable tool for educators who are using healthcare simulation. By understanding the different learning theories and how they can be applied, educators can design tailored learning activities that are effective and efficient for a particular student population.

References

Clapper, T. C. (2010). Beyond Knowles: What those conducting simulation need to know about adult learning theory. *Clinical Simulation in Nursing, 6*(1), e7–e14. https://doi.org/10.1016/j. ecns.2009.07.003

Kirkpatrick, D., & Kirkpatrick, J. (2006). *Evaluating training programs: The four levels.* Berrett-Koehler Publishers.

Knowles, M. S. (1980). *The modern practice of adult education: From pedagogy to andragogy.* Association Press.

Kolb, D. (1984). *Experiential learning: Experience as the source of learning and development* (Vol. 1).

Krathwohl, D. R. (2002). A revision of Bloom's taxonomy: An overview. *Theory Practice, 41*(4), 212–218.

Mcleod, S. (2022, November 3). Kolb's learning styles & experiential learning cycle. Accessed September 17, 2023. https://www.simplypsychology.org/learning-kolb.html

Miller, G. E. (1990). The assessment of clinical skills/competence/performance. *Academic Medicine, 65*(9), S63.

Chapter 3
The Learning Contract in Healthcare Simulation

Abstract This chapter underscores the pivotal role of learning contracts in healthcare simulation, emphasizing their significance in cultivating trust and respect between faculty and participants. Learning contracts serve as agreements outlining simulation expectations, goals, roles, and rules, fostering a safe and supportive learning environment. By providing clarity on learning objectives, specific assessment criteria, and acknowledging the simulated nature of the environment, educators can enhance engagement, reduce stress, and promote effective communication. The chapter also highlights the vital contribution of simulation programs in supporting learning contracts, emphasizing elements such as scheduling, process orientation, confidentiality, and grading policies. Overall, learning contracts prove to be invaluable tools, aligning educators, learners, and simulation programs in achieving meaningful engagement and learning outcomes in healthcare simulation.

Keywords Learning contracts · Simulation expectations · Safe learning environment · Effective communication · Engagement · Trust

3.1 Why Should We Have Learning Contracts?

Healthcare simulation is valuable for training healthcare professionals in a safe and controlled environment. However, the success of simulation programs depends on the relationship between faculty and participants. This relationship must be built on trust and respect and should be designed to promote learning and growth (Hughes & Hughes, 2023; Phrampus, 2019; Rudolph et al., 2014).

Learning contracts in healthcare simulation, also known as fiction contracts, can be a powerful tool for building relationships and promoting learning. A learning contract is an agreement (either verbal or written) between the learner and the instructor that outlines the expectations for the simulation, including the goals of the simulation, the roles that learners will play, and the rules that will be followed (Fig. 3.1).

Benefits of using learning contracts in healthcare simulation include:

Fig. 3.1 Learning contract

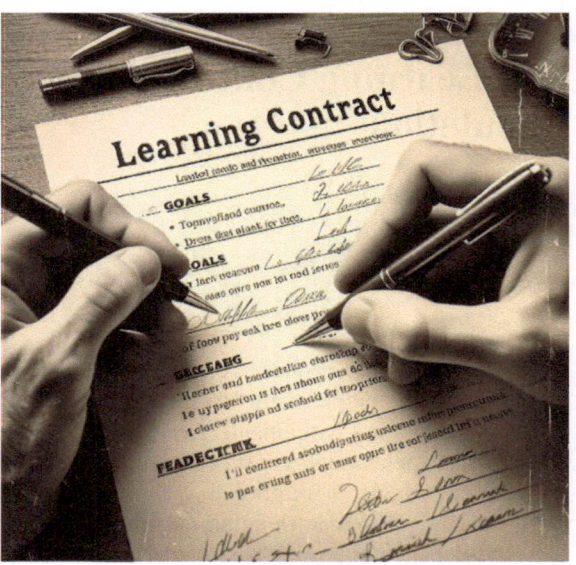

- **Promotes a safe and supportive learning environment**: The learning contract promotes a safe and supportive learning environment by establishing clear expectations and boundaries.
- **Improves learning**: When learners know what they are trying to learn and how they will be assessed, they are more likely to be engaged in the learning process.
- **Enhances engagement**: The learning contract can help learners become more engaged in the simulation by creating a sense of purpose and ownership over their learning.
- **Time value**: By focusing on the learner's specific learning goals, the instructor and learner can save time on activities irrelevant to the learner's needs.
- **Promotes communication**: The learning contract provides a clear framework for communication about the learner's learning goals, progress and expectations.
- **Reduces stress**: Knowing what learners need to do to succeed in simulation can help to reduce stress and anxiety.

3.2 How to Make an Effective Learning Contract?

Here are some tips for simulation educators on how to use learning contracts to build relationships and promote learning in healthcare simulation (Hughes & Hughes, 2023; Phrampus, 2019; Rudolph et al., 2014):

- Be clear and **transparent about the learning objectives** and expectations for each simulation.

- Establish clear and **specific assessment criteria** for each learning outcome. This will ensure learners know what they need to do to demonstrate mastery of the objective.
- Acknowledge that simulation is **not real** but indicate that the simulation will be "real enough" to create a successful learning environment.
- Ensure we are **not here to deliberately trick** learners or to make them feel bad about themselves. Instead, our goals are to help learners identify and address their individual learning needs.
- Promote a safe and supportive learning environment. Let learners know that it is **okay to make mistakes** in simulation and that the goal is to learn from them.
- Convey the message that the simulation educator is **here to help** learners achieve their learning goals and be a better version of them.
- Emphasize the importance of **meaningful use of time**. Ensure that the program's content is carefully crafted to meet the needs of their learning cohort in a timely manner.

3.3 Role of the Simulation Program in Support of Learning Contracts

The Learning Contract is important to the entire simulation program, not just simulation educators as the learning contract helps to ensure learner engagement. Thus, the simulation program has a vital role in supporting the learning contract, including:

- **Schedule**: The simulation program should provide learners with a clear understanding of the time commitment required for the simulation, including the sequence of events and the time allotted for each activity.
- **Process orientation**: The simulation program should provide learners with an orientation to the simulation process, including what happens during the simulation, whether learners can talk to faculty during the simulation, whether debriefing will occur afterward, and whether there will be time for questions and answers.
- **Learning materials**: The simulation program provides learners access to case studies and other pre-simulation learning materials. This will help learners to prepare for the simulation and to develop the knowledge and skills they need to be successful.
- **Equipment and environment**: The simulation program should provide learners with proper orientation to the equipment and the care environment that will be used during the simulation. This may include training on how to use specific equipment and familiarizing learners with the layout and features of the simulation environment.
- **Confidentiality**: The simulation program should pledge to protect learners' performance data privacy. This means the simulation program should not share learners' performance data with anyone without their permission. This includes

adopting a video use policy. If the simulation program intends to use video recordings of learners, it should have a clear video use policy that explains how the recordings will be used and stored.

- **Grading policies**: The simulation program should have clear grading policies in place for simulation activities. This includes specifying how learners will be assessed and what criteria will be used to determine grades. Further, an understanding of whether the grades are formative (for progression) or summative (as a final grade) is critical.

Overall, learning contracts are valuable tools for promoting meaningful engagement and learning in healthcare simulation. By using learning contracts, instructors can help learners to achieve their learning goals and to develop the skills and knowledge they need to provide safe and effective care.

References

Hughes, P. G., & Hughes, K. E. (2023). Briefing prior to simulation activity. In: *StatPearls*. StatPearls Publishing. Accessed September 26, 2023. http://www.ncbi.nlm.nih.gov/books/NBK545234/

Phrampus, P. E. (2019, July 23). 5 elements in my approach to the learning contract in simulation. *Simulating healthcare*. A blog dedicated to discussions and relevant things regarding simulation in healthcare. Accessed September 25, 2023. https://simulatinghealthcare.net/2019/07/23/5-elements-in-my-approach-to-the-learning-contract-in-simulation/

Rudolph, J. W., Raemer, D. B., & Simon, R. (2014). Establishing a safe container for learning in simulation: The role of the presimulation briefing. *Journal of the Society for Simulation in Healthcare, 9*(6), 339–349. https://doi.org/10.1097/SIH.0000000000000047

Chapter 4
Healthcare Simulation Modalities

Abstract This chapter delves into the diverse landscape of healthcare simulation modalities, categorizing them into two primary types: physical simulation and digital simulation. Physical simulation includes task trainers, manikins, and standardized patients, each offering distinct advantages and disadvantages. Task trainers, cost-effective and portable, excel in specific skill practice. Manikins, ranging from low to high fidelity, simulate various patients for comprehensive training. Standardized patients, skilled actors representing patients, enhance communication and examination skills. The digital realm introduces extended reality (XR) modalities, including virtual reality (VR), augmented reality (AR), and mixed reality (MR). These digital simulations enable immersive, safe, and versatile training experiences. The chapter explores the benefits and applications of each modality, emphasizing the importance of aligning the choice with learning objectives, resource availability, and learner needs.

Keywords Physical simulation · Digital simulation · Task trainers · Manikins · Simulation modalities

Healthcare simulation modalities can roughly be divided into two main categories: physical simulation and digital simulation. Physical simulation modalities include task trainers, manikins, and standardized patients. Extended Reality (XR) or Digital simulation modalities include virtual reality (VR), augmented reality (AR), and mixed reality (MR) (https://www.qualcomm.com/research/extended-reality; Kardong-Edgren et al., 2022; Lopreiato et al., 2016; Verkuyl et al., 2022). Each simulation modality has its advantages and disadvantages (Datta et al., 2012). For example, task trainers are relatively inexpensive and easy to use, but they may not be as realistic as other modalities. Manikins can be very realistic, but they can be more expensive and difficult to transport. Standardized patients can provide real-time feedback, but they can be variable in their performance depending on the thoroughness of their training and preparation.

The choice of simulation modality will depend on a number of factors, including the learning objectives, the resources available, and the learner's needs. By carefully

T. Tangpaisarn et al., *Navigating Healthcare Simulation*,
SpringerBriefs in Education, https://doi.org/10.1007/978-3-031-81265-1_4

choosing the suitable simulation modality, educators can help learners to develop the skills and knowledge they need to provide safe and effective care.

4.1   Task Trainers

Task trainers are specialized simulators or lifelike models of human body parts designed to help learners practice a specific skill. They are typically made of plastic or silicone and can be quite realistic. Task trainers are a good option for practicing skills that are difficult to practice on actual patients (Singh & Restivo, 2023).

Examples of Task Trainers

- **Airway task trainer**: An airway task trainer is a model of a patient's head and neck that learners can use to practice airway management skills, such as intubation and suctioning. It typically has a realistic airway anatomy and can be used to simulate various airway conditions (Fig. 4.1).
- **Suture trainer**: A suture trainer is a model of a wound that learners can use to practice suturing. It typically has a rubber base and a silicone skin that can be cut and sutured.
- **IV insertion trainer**: An IV insertion trainer is a model of an arm that learners can use to practice IV insertion. It typically has a vein that can be palpated and punctured.
- **Catheterization trainer**: A catheterization trainer is a model of a pelvis that learners can use to practice catheterization. It typically has a urethra that can be catheterized.

Benefits of Using Task Trainers in Healthcare Simulation

- **Safety**: Task trainers allow learners to practice skills without the risk of harming a real patient.
- **Feedback**: Task trainers can be used to provide feedback to learners on their performance.
- **Accessibility**: Task trainers are relatively inexpensive and easy to obtain.
- **Portability**: Task trainers are typically portable, making them easy to use in various settings.

4.2   Manikins

While some medical professionals still refer to these training devices as "mannequins," the preferred term is manikin. This is because research publications, professional associations, and suppliers are increasingly using the term manikin. The word "mannequin" is also regarded to be more closely associated with the

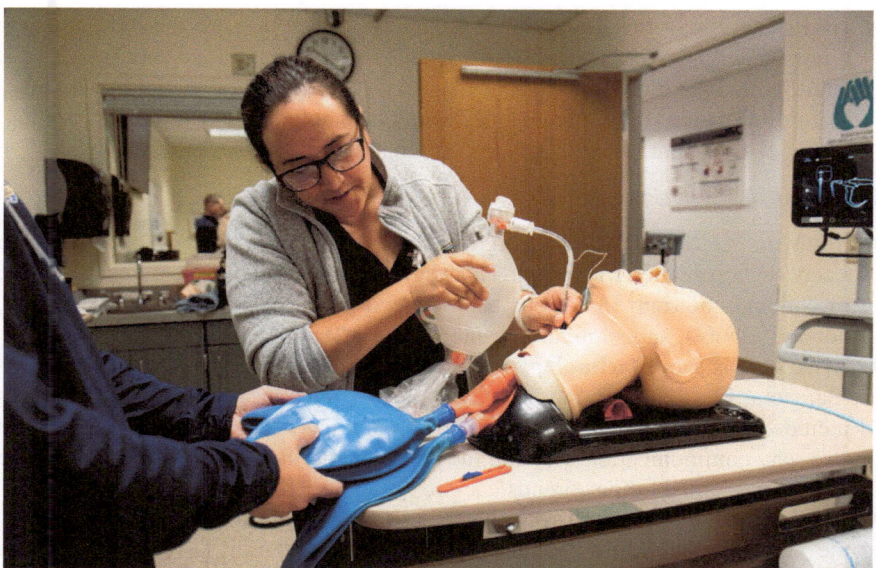

Fig. 4.1 Airway task trainer (*photo courtesy* WISER)

fashion industry rather than with healthcare (https://www.healthysimulation.com/manikin/). Manikins are life-sized devices that can be used to simulate a variety of different patients. They are typically made of plastic or silicone and can be quite realistic. Manikins are used to train healthcare professionals in various skills, including physical examination, assessment, and treatment. Computerized manikins can be programmed to respond to certain stimuli, such as pain or medication administration, and can provide feedback to learners on their performance through integrated software that can display realistic physiologic responses.

Types of Manikins

Manikins can be classified into three main types based on their level of technology. The simulation industry often misuses the word fidelity which leads to confusion in terms of the expected capabilities of manikins (https://www.healthysimulation.com/manikin/; Meerdink & Khan, 2021; Torres et al., 2022).

- **Low-technology manikins**: Low-**technology** manikins are typically used to teach basic skills, such as CPR and IV insertion. They are often made of plastic or rubber and have a limited range of features.
- **Mid-technology manikins**: Mid-**technology** manikins are more realistic than low-technology manikins and can teach a broader range of skills, such as advanced cardiac life support and airway management. They typically have more advanced features, such as a pulse, breath sounds, and pupils that dilate and constrict.

- **High-technology manikins**: High-**technology** manikins are the most realistic type of manikin and can be used to teach more complex skills, such as critical care and trauma care management. They typically include all of the mid-technology features as well as a wider range of capabilities including a heartbeat, breathing, and vital signs that can be monitored and manipulated.

Examples of Manikins

- **SimMan 3G**: SimMan 3G is a high-**technology** manikin that is produced by the Laerdal® corporation (Stavanger, Norway). It can be used to simulate a wide range of patient conditions in various healthcare settings, including medical schools, nursing schools, and simulation centers (Fig. 4.2).
- **Ares**: Ares is a mid-**technology** manikin that is produced by Elevate Healthcare® (Sarasota, FL, USA) formerly known as CAE Healthcare®. Practical features include muscle injection sites, a realistic breathing system, a difficult airway, and two-way communication between the manikin and the student (https://www.cae healthcare.com/solutions/brands/cae-ares/).
- **Noelle**: Noelle is a high-**technology** birthing manikin that is produced by the Gaumard Scientific® (Miami, FL, USA). It is used to teach healthcare professionals how to manage childbirth and other obstetric emergencies.

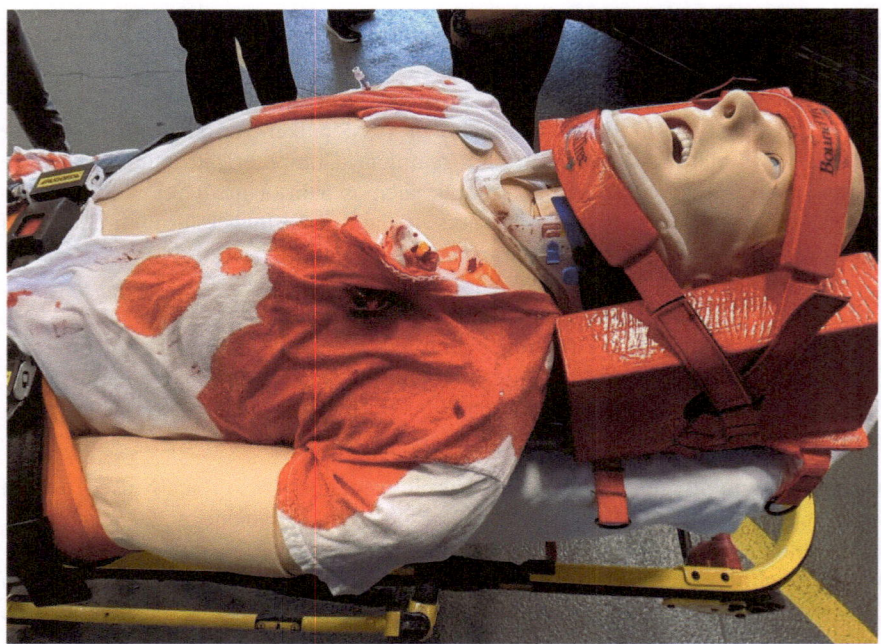

Fig. 4.2 High-technology Laerdal® SimMan 3G manikin (*photo courtesy* WISER)

Benefits of Using Manikins in Healthcare Simulation

- **Patient Safety**: Manikins allow learners to practice clinical skills in a safe environment without the risk of harming a real patient.
- **Realism**: Manikins can be very realistic, which can help learners develop the skills and knowledge they need to provide safe and effective care in real-world settings. We can enhance the realism of manikins by adding Moulage and other props—including wigs or clothing.
- **Engagement**: Manikins can be engaging and motivating for learners by providing cues as to a patient's state through the demonstration of vital signs such as pupil dilation, rate of pulse, rate of breath through chest rise and fall, or circulation through cyanotic discoloration.
- **Affordability**: Depending on their acquisition cost, long-term durability and other factors such as the availability of the actual clinical experience, manikins can be a cost-effective way to train healthcare professionals.

4.3   Standardized Patients

Standardized patients (SPs) are people who are trained to act as patients in simulated scenarios. They are typically used to practice communication skills, patient education, and physical examination. SPs can provide feedback on the learner's performance and can help them to identify areas where they need to improve.

SPs are trained to portray a variety of different patients with different ages, genders, and medical conditions. They are also trained to respond to a variety of different stimuli, such as questions from the learner or physical examination findings. In the design of simulation scenarios, SP levels of skill can range from that of highly trained professionals with very scripted responses to peers engaged in playing a role within the scenario (https://www.midwestern.edu/campus-life/glenda e-az-campus/campus-facilities/clinical-skills-and-simulation-center/standardi zed-patient-program; https://www.omed.pitt.edu/sp-program/for-prospective-sps; https://www.utsouthwestern.edu/departments/simulation-center/services/standardi zed-patient/faq.html; Shankar & Dwivedi, 2016; Uzelli Yılmaz et al., 2022).

Examples of Skills that Can Be Targeted with SP Utilization

- **Communication skills**: SPs can be used to teach learners how to communicate effectively with patients or colleagues.
- **Patient education**: SPs can be used to teach learners how to educate patients about their medical conditions and treatment plans (Fig. 4.3).
- **Physical examination**: SPs can be used to teach learners how to perform a physical examination.

Benefits of Using SPs in Healthcare Simulation

- **Realism**: SPs can provide a very realistic learning experience for students.

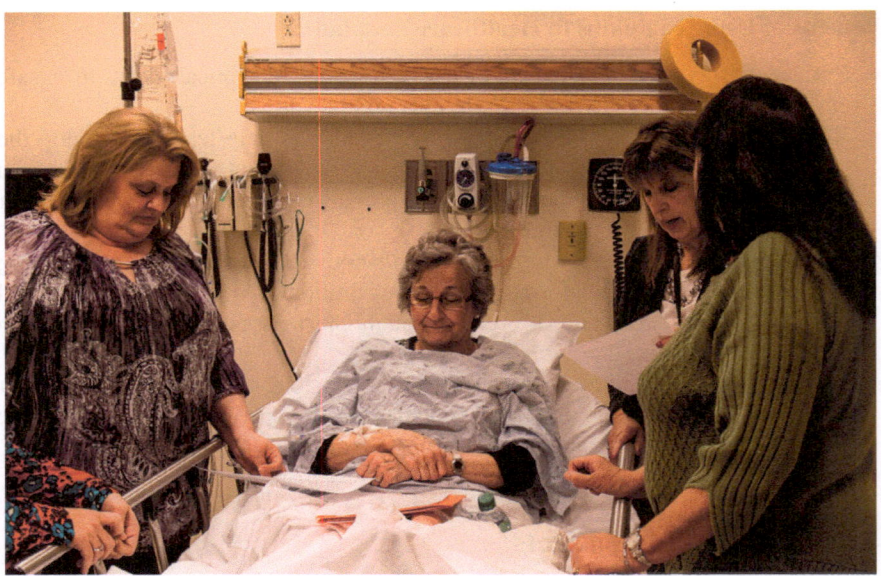

Fig. 4.3 Assessment performed on standardized patient (*photo courtesy* WISER)

- **Versatility**: SPs can be used to simulate a variety of different patients with different ages, genders, and medical conditions.
- **Feedback**: SPs can provide feedback to learners on their performance.

Tips for Using SPs in Healthcare Simulation

- **Clear instruction**: The SP should be thoroughly briefed about the simulation design, be familiar with the role they are playing and be informed of the goals of the simulation.
- **Provide learner feedback**: The SP can be prepared to provide feedback to the learner on their performance during and after the simulation.
- **Dignity and Respect**: It is important to recognize that the SP is a professional, should be treated with respect and allowed to maintain their personal dignity. This is critical as SPs are often being physically examined by multiple students during a simulation activity.

4.4 Hybrid Simulation

Hybrid simulation is a type of healthcare simulation that combines two or more simulation modalities. Commonly, hybrid simulation is defined as the utilization of wearable task trainer, or augmentative technology in conjunction with a human actor in a healthcare education context. (Brown & Tortorella, 2020; Lateef & Too, 2019)

The technology is typically used to simulate aspects of a particular medical scenario or intervention (such as invasive procedures) that would place an SP at risk (Brown & Tortorella, 2020).

Examples of Hybrid Simulation

- **Management of the patient with bacterial meningitis**: The SP would present with symptoms of bacterial meningitis, such as headache, fever, stiff neck, and confusion. Learners would be responsible for conducting a physical examination, obtaining a history, and performing a lumbar puncture to collect cerebrospinal fluid (CSF). The lumbar puncture simulator would allow learners to practice the procedure in a safe and controlled environment while still permitting them to communicate with the SP portraying an infected patient.
- **Venipuncture in the COVID-19 pandemic**: Learners can practice venipuncture while communicating with the SP portraying a patient with COVID-19 in a negative pressure room (Fig. 4.4).
- **Obstetric emergency management**: The SP or manikin would wear a Mama Natalie birthing simulator. The Mama Natalie (Laerdal Corp., Stavanger, Norway) birthing simulator would allow learners to practice managing obstetric emergencies, such as shoulder dystocia, postpartum hemorrhage, and breech presentation, while affording the opportunity to communicate with an SP portraying a parturient.

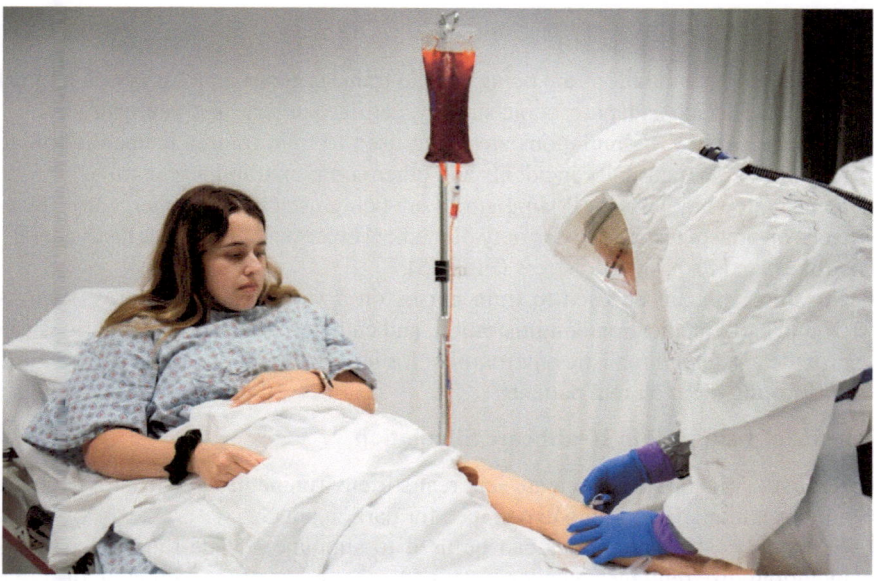

Fig. 4.4 Venipuncture training in the COVID-19 pandemic (*photo courtesy* WISER)

Benefits of Using Hybrid Simulations in Healthcare Simulation

- **Realism**: Hybrid simulation can combine the benefits of different simulation modalities to create a more comprehensive learning experience. The increased realism can help the learner to better understand how the simulation connects to actual clinical care without risk of harm to the SP.
- **Wide range of skills**: Hybrid simulation can be used to train for a wide range of skills, including technical and non-technical (e.g. communication, decision-making, leadership, care coordination, delegation) simultaneously.

4.5 Virtual Reality (VR)

Virtual reality (VR) is a **computer-simulated environment** that can be used to create realistic scenarios for learner practice. VR simulations can be used to practice a wide range of skills, including surgery, trauma care, emergency medicine, and nursing. VR simulations are beneficial for practicing skills that are difficult or dangerous to practice in a real-world setting (https://www.umaryland.edu/fctl/resources/technology/emerging-trends/virtual-reality-vr/; Pottle, 2019; https://www.healthysimulation.com/virtual-reality-in-medicine).

VR simulations work by using a headset to create a computer-generated image that the user sees as if it were the real world. The user can then interact with the virtual environment using hand controllers or virtual devices.

Examples of VR

- **Surgery**: VR simulations are being used to train surgeons on a variety of surgical procedures, such as laparoscopic surgery, cardiac surgery, and neurosurgery.
- **Trauma care**: VR simulations are being used to train trauma teams on how to respond to mass casualty incidents and other complex trauma scenarios.
- **Emergency medicine**: VR simulations are being used to train emergency physicians on how to respond to a variety of medical emergencies, such as heart attacks, strokes, and respiratory distress (Fig. 4.5).
- **Nursing**: VR can be used to train nurses on a variety of procedures, such as wound care, medication administration, and catheterization. VR simulations can provide a safe and realistic environment for nurses to practice these skills before performing them on real patients.

Benefits of Using VR in Healthcare Simulation

- **Realism**: VR simulations create very realistic environments, which helps to create a more immersive learning experience for participants.
- **Versatility**: VR simulations can be used to simulate a wide range of patients including different ages, genders and medical conditions, as well as in different environment
- **Safety**: VR simulations allow learners to practice skills in a safe and controlled environment without the risk of harming themselves or a real patient.

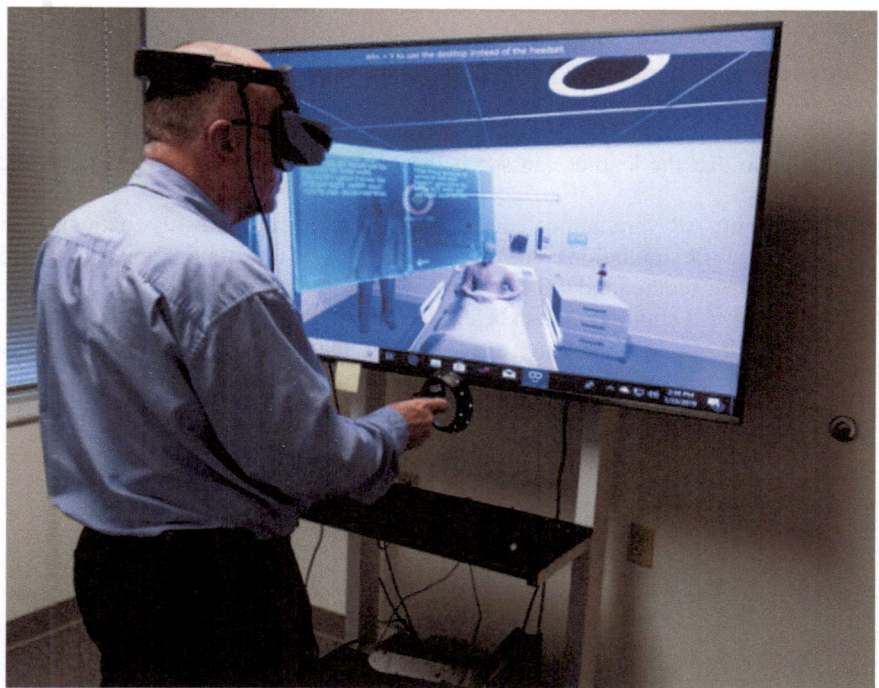

Fig. 4 5 Virtual reality training (*photo* courtesy WISER)

- **Engagement**: VR simulations can be engaging and motivating for learners.
- **Distance learning**: VR can facilitate collaborative learning experiences, even in remote or distributed settings. Learners can gather in a shared virtual environment, conduct group discussions, or work together on problem-solving tasks.

4.6 Augmented Reality (AR)

Augmented reality (AR) is a technology that **overlays** digital information onto physical objects in the real world. AR simulations can be used to provide learners with information and feedback while they are practicing skills on physical simulation modalities. AR simulations are beneficial for training new learners or learners who are practicing complex skills (Dhar et al., 2021; Gerup et al., 2020; https://www.healthysimulation.com/virtual-reality-in-medicine/).

AR simulations work by using a camera to capture the real world and then overlaying digital information on the image. The user can then see the digital information superimposed on the real world.

Examples of AR

- **Physical examination**: AR simulations can be used to provide learners with real-time feedback on their physical examination skills. For example, an AR simulation could overlay the image of a patient's anatomy onto the learner's view of the real patient, so that the learner can see if they are palpating the correct anatomical structures.
- **Assessment**: AR simulations can be used to help learners assess patients. For example, an AR simulation could overlay the image of ultrasonography performed by the learner on the model (Fig. 4.6).
- **Treatment**: AR simulations can be used to help learners practice treatment skills. For example, an AR simulation could overlay the image of a patient's anatomy onto the learner's view of the real patient so that the learner can see if they are performing a procedure correctly.

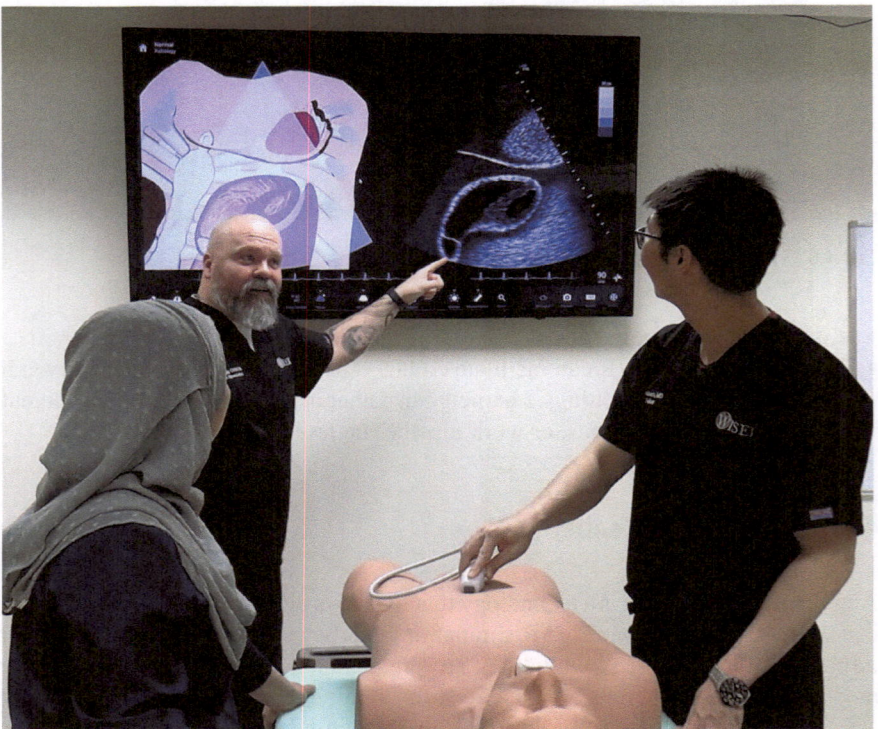

Fig. 4.6 Augmented reality imaging while utilizing the Vimedix ultrasound simulator (Elevate Healthcare®, Sarasota, Fl., USA) (*photo courtesy* WISER)

Benefits of Using AR Simulations in Healthcare Simulation

- **Quality and safety**: AR can be used to overlay 3D anatomical information onto a patient, allowing learners to see the patient's anatomy in real-time. This can help to improve the accuracy of procedures and reduce the risk of complications.
- **Reduced costs**: AR can eliminate the need for redundant screens, as all imaging and patient data can be integrated into a single AR display. This can save hospitals money on equipment costs.
- **Realism**: AR can be used to create immersive and realistic training simulations. This can help medical professionals to more effectively learn new procedures and improve their skills.

4.7 Mixed Reality (MR)

Mixed reality (MR) is a technology that combines virtual reality (VR) and augmented reality (AR). MR simulations allow learners to interact with both the virtual and real worlds simultaneously. MR is a step beyond AR, but it retains elements of the user's real world. AR enhances a viewer's perspective of the real world, while MR blurs the difference between the real world and virtual world. VR does not retain any features of the real-world surroundings. MR simulations are beneficial for training learners on complex skills that require them to interact with both the virtual and real worlds.

MR simulations work by using a headset to create a computer-generated image that the user sees as if it were the real world. The user can then interact with the virtual environment using hand controllers or other devices. The headset also uses cameras to capture the real world and then overlay digital information on the image. The user can then see the digital information superimposed on the real world (Gerup et al., 2020; https://www.simxvr.com/glossary/mixed-reality-definition/).

Examples of MR

- **MR-guided subclavian venous access (SVA)**: A virtual needle is overlaid on the patient's real-time ultrasound image, guiding the clinician to the correct insertion point for the SVA catheter (Robinson et al., 2014).
- **MR-enhanced surgical training**: MR images can be used to create a virtual model of a joint, which can then be used to practice joint replacement surgery.
- **Obstetric MR**: By synchronizing holograms with the physical world, Obstetric MR allows learners to see inside manikin and observe the dynamic physiology underlying difficult deliveries to promote deeper learning (https://www.gaumard.com/obstetricmr) (Fig. 4.7).

Benefits of Using MR Simulations in Healthcare Simulation

- **Realism**: MR simulations can create very realistic environments, which can help to create a more immersive learning experience for learners.

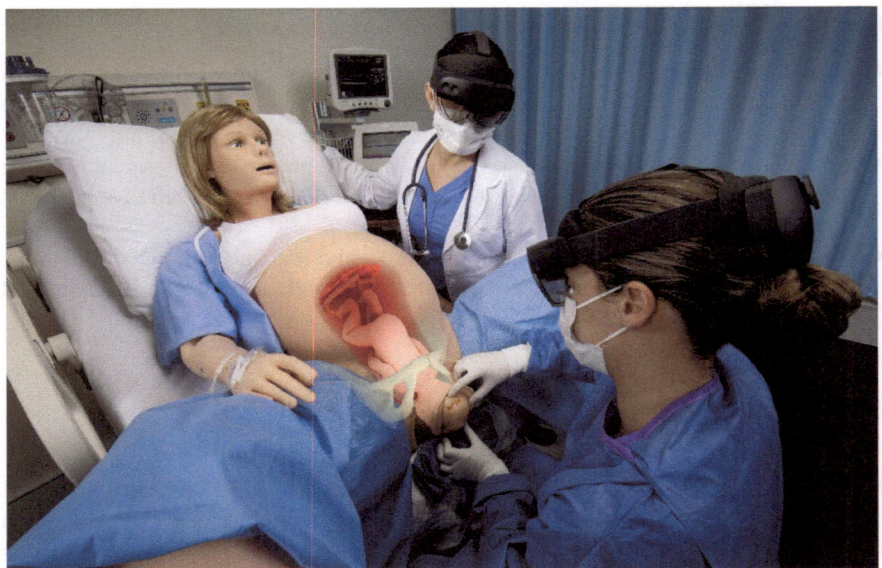

Fig. 4.7 Mixed reality—mixed reality training in obstetric care (VICTORIA® S2200) (*photo courtesy* Gaumard® Scientific, Miami, FL, USA)

- **Interactivity**: MR simulations allow learners to interact with both the virtual and real worlds simultaneously, which can help them develop the skills they need to provide safe and effective care in a real-world setting.

VR, AR, and MR simulations are relatively new technologies in healthcare simulation, but they can potentially revolutionize how healthcare professionals are trained. By using these modalities, educators can increase learner engagement and help them to develop the knowledge and skills needed to provide safe and effective care.

4.8   Summary

The best simulation modality for a particular learner or learning objective will depend on several factors, including the skill being practiced, the learner's level of experience, and the resources available. Task trainers are a good option for practicing specific skills that are difficult to practice on real patients. Manikins are a good option for practicing a wide range of skills, including physical examination, assessment, and treatment. Standardized patients or SPs are a good option for practicing communication skills, patient education, and physical examination. VR, AR, and MR simulations are good options for practicing skills that are difficult or dangerous to practice in a real-world setting. Hybrid simulations can be used to create very realistic and challenging scenarios for learner practice.

Simulation educators should carefully consider the learner's needs and the learning objectives when choosing a simulation modality. By using the most effective simulation modality, educators can help learners to develop the skills and knowledge they need to provide safe and effective care.

References

Augmented Reality in Medicine | Healthcare Simulation | HealthySimulation.com. Published May 29, 2019. Accessed October 19, 2023. https://www.healthysimulation.com/augmented-reality-in-medicine/

Brown, W. J., & Tortorella, R. A. W. (2020). Hybrid medical simulation—A systematic literature review. *Smart Learning Environments, 7*(1), 16. https://doi.org/10.1186/s40561-020-00127-6

CAE Healthcare—Meet CAE Ares. CAE Healthcare. Accessed October 20, 2023. https://www.cae healthcare.com/solutions/brands/cae-ares/

Datta, R., Upadhyay, K., & Jaideep, C. (2012). Simulation and its role in medical education. *Medical Journal of Armed Forces India, 68*(2), 167–172. https://doi.org/10.1016/S0377-1237(12)600 40-9

Dhar, P., Rocks, T., Samarasinghe, R.M., Stephenson, G., & Smith, C. (2021) Augmented reality in medical education: Students' experiences and learning outcomes. *Medical Education Online, 26*(1), 1953953. https://doi.org/10.1080/10872981.2021.1953953

Extended Reality XR | Immersive VR | Qualcomm. Accessed October 17, 2023. https://www.qua lcomm.com/research/extended-reality

For Prospective Standardized/Simulated Patients | Office of Medical Education, School of Medicine | University of Pittsburgh. Accessed October 2, 2023. https://www.omed.pitt.edu/sp-program/for-prospective-sps

Gerup, J., Soerensen, C. B., & Dieckmann, P. (2020). Augmented reality and mixed reality for healthcare education beyond surgery: An integrative review. *International Journal of Medical Education, 11*, 1–18. https://doi.org/10.5116/ijme.5e01.eb1a

Kardong-Edgren, S., Swiderski, D., Noland, H., Wasseem, M., Charles, S., & Chen, S. (2022) *CHSE blueprint review reference manual.* Society for Simulation in Healthcare.

Latee, F., & Too, X. Y. (2019). The 2019 WACEM expert document on hybrid simulation for transforming health-care simulation through mixing and matching. *Journal of Emergencies, Trauma, and Shock, 12*(4), 243–247. https://doi.org/10.4103/JETS.JETS_112_19

Lopreiato, J. O., Downing, D., Gammon, W., et al. (2016). Healthcare Simulation Dictionary. http://www.ssih.org/dictionary

Manikin | Manikins vs. Mannequins | Healthcare Simulation | HealthySimulation.com. Published May 5, 2012. Accessed October 2, 2023. https://www.healthysimulation.com/manikin/

Meerdink, M., & Khan, J. (2021). Comparison of the use of manikins and simulated patients in a multidisciplinary in situ medical simulation program for healthcare professionals in the United Kingdom. *Journal of Educational Evaluation for Health Professions, 18*, 8. https://doi.org/10.3352/jeehp.2021.18.8

Obstetric MR^{TM} | Mixed Reality Enhanced Learning System. Accessed January 29, 2024. https://www.gaumard.com/obstetricmr

Pottle, J. (2019). Virtual reality and the transformation of medical education. *Future Healthcare Journal, 6*(3), 181–185. https://doi.org/10.7861/fhj.2019-0036

Robinson, A. R., Gravenstein, N., Cooper, L. A., Lizdas, D., Luria, I., & Lampotang, S. (2014). A mixed-reality part-task trainer for subclavian venous access. *Journal of Society Simulation in Healthcare, 9*(1), 56–64. https://doi.org/10.1097/SIH.0b013e31829b3fb3

Shankar, P. R., & Dwivedi, N. R. (2016). Standardized patient's views about their role in the teaching-learning process of undergraduate basic science medical students. *Journal of Clinical and Diagnostic Research: JCDR*, *10*(6):JC01-JC05. https://doi.org/10.7860/JCDR/2016/18827. 7944

Standardized Patient Program Frequently Asked Questions. Accessed October 18, 2023. https:// www.utsouthwestern.edu/departments/simulation-center/services/standardized-patient/faq. html

Singh, M., & Restivo, A. (2023) Task trainers in procedural skills acquisition in medical simulation. In: *StatPearls*. StatPearls Publishing. Accessed October 2, 2023. http://www.ncbi.nlm.nih.gov/ books/NBK558925/

Standardized Patient Program. Accessed October 18, 2023. https://www.midwestern.edu/campus-life/glendale-az-campus/campus-facilities/clinical-skills-and-simulation-center/standardized-patient-program

Torres, K., Evans, P., Mamcarz, I., Radczuk, N., & Torres, A. (2022). A manikin or human simulator—development of a tool for measuring students' perception. *PeerJ, 10*, e14214. https://doi. org/10.7717/peerj.14214

University of Maryland, Baltimore. Virtual Reality (VR). Accessed October 19, 2023. https://www. umaryland.edu/fctl/resources/technology/emerging-trends/virtual-reality-vr/

Uzelli Yılmaz, D., Last, N., Harvey, J., Norman, L., Monteiro, S., & Sibbald, M. (2022). Quality in standardized patient training and delivery: Retrospective documentary analysis of trainer and instructor feedback. *Cureus, 14*(1), e21022. https://doi.org/10.7759/cureus.21022

Verkuyl, M., Taplay, K., Atack, L., et al. (2022, February 28). Technological variety. Accessed October 2, 2023. https://ecampusontario.pressbooks.pub/vlsvstoolkit/chapter/technological-var iety-in-virtual-simulation/

Virtual Reality in Medicine | Healthcare Simulation | HealthySimulation.com. Published August 1, 2019. Accessed October 18, 2023. https://www.healthysimulation.com/virtual-reality-in-med icine/

What Is Mixed Reality? Virtual Reality Medical Simulation | SimX. Accessed October 19, 2023. https://www.simxvr.com/glossary/mixed-reality-definition/

Chapter 5
Simulation Locale

Abstract In this comprehensive exploration of healthcare simulation locales, the study delineates four primary settings for simulation-based medical education: simulation centers, in-situ environments, mobile units, and ad hoc or off-site locations. Simulation centers, dedicated facilities equipped with high-fidelity mannequins and experienced staff, offer a controlled environment for a broad spectrum of medical training. In-situ simulation, conducted within actual clinical settings, enhances realism, teamwork, and hazard identification but may disrupt patient care. Mobile unit simulation brings training to underserved areas, though with limited capacity. Ad hoc simulation, in non-traditional settings, provides accessibility but requires careful logistics coordination. The choice of locale hinges on factors such as learning objectives, target audience, and available resources, each option presenting unique advantages and challenges. Considerations for successful in-situ simulation implementation are outlined, underscoring the importance of meticulous planning and collaboration with relevant stakeholders.

Keywords Simulation centers · In-situ simulation · Mobile unit simulation · Ad hoc simulation · Simulation location

Healthcare simulation locale refers to the physical environment in which simulation-based medical education takes place. The four main types of healthcare simulation locales are simulation centers, in-situ, mobile units, and ad hoc, or off-site locations. The choice of healthcare simulation locale depends on a number of factors, including the learning objectives of the simulation, the target audience, the available resources, and the potential benefits and drawbacks of each setting.

5.1 Simulation Centers

Simulation center can vary in terms of size, complexity and capabilities. Some centers can be large, purpose built and comprehensive while others occupy a small part of the hospital that has converted space to be used for simulation-based training purposes. Some hospital departments provide off-site simulation as in-house training room (s) specifically set up for simulation training away from the clinical setting but within a hospital department (Sørensen et al., 2017). For example, at the Winter Institute for Simulation, Education, and Research (WISER), we have one main simulation center as the headquarters with 12, smaller satellite centers located physically in various hospitals and schools. Simulation centers are dedicated facilities that are designed for healthcare simulation. They typically have a variety of simulation rooms that are equipped with high-technology mannequins, task trainers, complex audio/ visual systems and a wide range of support equipment. Simulation centers also have experienced staff who can facilitate simulations and provide feedback to learners.

Simulation centers can be used to train healthcare professionals in a wide range of skills, including:

- Basic clinical procedures, such as venipuncture, suturing, and catheterization
- Complex team-based scenarios, such as code blues, traumatic injuries, and obstetric emergencies
- Communication and teamwork skills
- Patient safety and risk management skills
- Leadership and decision-making skills.

Depending on the mission of the program Simulation centers may be used by a variety of healthcare professionals, including physicians, nurses, paramedics, and other allied health professionals. Other simulation centers are created and operated for specific learner groups, such as simulation programs within a school of nursing.

Examples of Simulation Center Training Programs

- Train a team of nurses on how to respond to a code blue (Fig. 5.1).
- Train a new surgeon on how to perform a complex surgical procedure.
- Train a medical student on how to manage a patient who has a critical condition.
- Train a nursing student on how to perform venipuncture.

Advantages of Simulation Centers

- **Dedicated-space**: Simulation centers have dedicated space for simulation-based education. This means learners can practice skills and learn from mistakes in a safe and controlled environment without disrupting patient care.
- **Specialized-equipment**: Simulation centers have specialized equipment for simulation-based education, such as high-technology mannequins, task trainers, and audiovisual equipment. This equipment can help to create a realistic learning environment for learners.

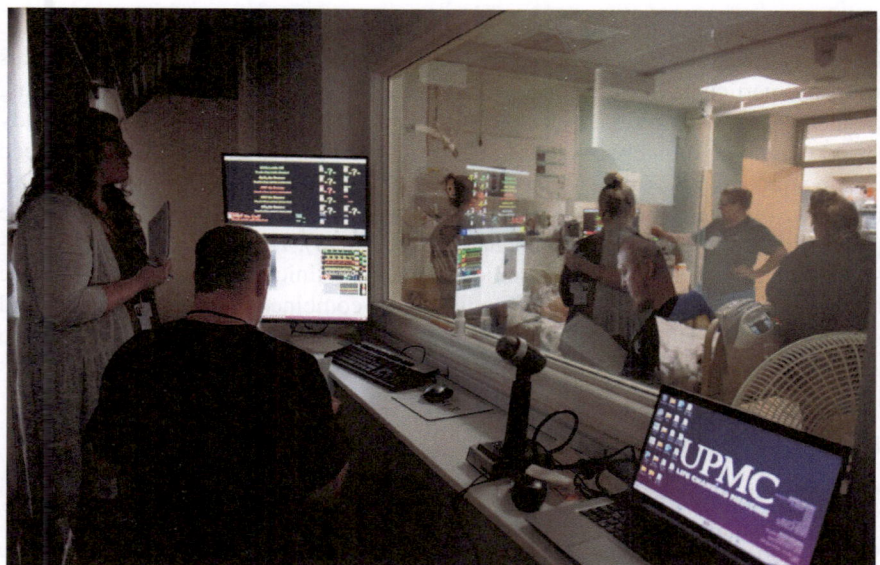

Fig. 5.1 Simulation center training exercise (*photo courtesy* WISER)

- **Experienced-staff**: Simulation centers have experienced staff who can assist in facilitating scenarios and assisting faculty/instructors to be able to provide feedback to learners. Working together, these teams can help learners to understand their mistakes, make needed corrections and thus improve their skills.

Disadvantages of Simulation Centers

- **Cost**: Simulation centers can be expensive to build and maintain.
- **Access**: Simulation centers may not be accessible to all healthcare professionals, especially those who work in rural or underserved areas.
- **Location**: The physical location of the simulation center may not be convenient to the learners.

5.2 In-Situ Simulation

In-situ simulation is a type of healthcare simulation that is conducted in the actual clinical setting where the skill or scenario being taught would be performed in real life. In-situ simulation is a relatively new type of simulation, but it is quickly becoming a popular training tool for healthcare professionals. In-situ simulation is an effective way to train learners in the most realistic of environments. This type of simulation is often used to uncover latent safety threats in clinical care areas. In-situ simulation can also be used to train teams on how to respond to emergencies in their workplace. In situ simulation can be conducted as either announced or unannounced. Both of these approaches have their own benefits and limitations. Some individuals who have participated in unannounced in-situ simulations describe it as intimidating (Anderson et al., 2005), but this topic is poorly explored in the literature. One study found that approximately one-third of all staff members thought that unannounced in-situ simulation was stressful and unpleasant, although all staff members before-hand had been told that a number of unannounced in-situ simulations would take place within a specific period (Sørensen et al., 2014). However, unannounced in-situ simulations offer a unique window on actual clinical care processes because the simulation-based educational activity can be combined with human factors and systems testing. This type of simulation has becoming increasingly important to ensure higher levels of provider and facility readiness for the increasingly ill patients being cared for in hospitals worldwide (Phrampus, 2014).

Examples of In-Situ Simulation

- A multidisciplinary team trained on how to respond to a deteriorating patient on the inpatient floor (Fig. 5.2).
- A group of physicians and nurses being prepared to manage a patient with malignant hyperthermia in the operating room.
- A multidisciplinary team on how to respond to a major trauma patient in the emergency department.

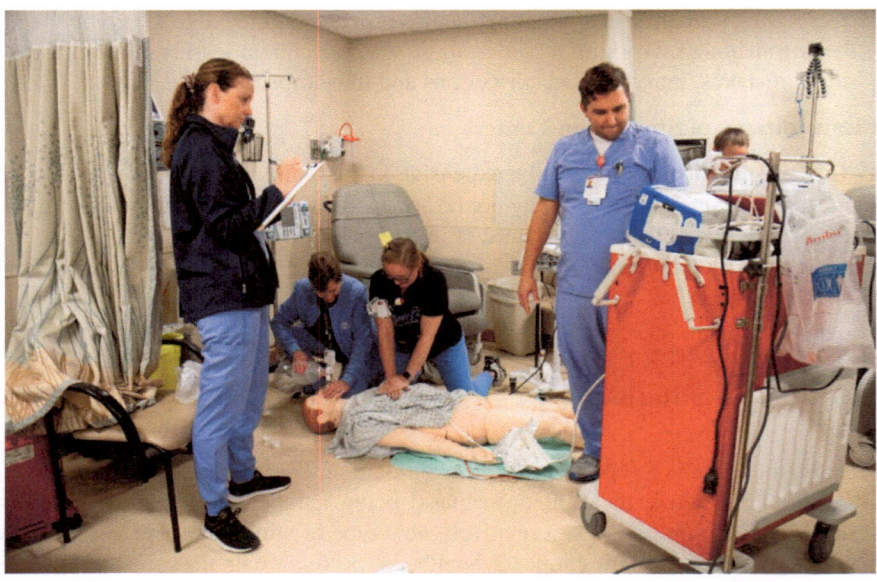

Fig. 5.2 In-situ simulation training for management of a patient found in cardiac arrest on a patient care unit (*photo courtesy* WISER)

Advantages of In-Situ Simulation

- **Increased realism**: In-situ simulation is more realistic than other types of simulation because it takes place in the actual patient care setting. This allows learners to practice skills and learn from mistakes in a safe, controlled yet highly realistic environment.
- **Easy to access**: In-situ simulation is easy for staff to attend and less disruptive to their schedules and other clinical responsibilities.
- **Improved teamwork and communication**: In-situ simulation can help to improve teamwork and communication among healthcare professionals. This is because in-situ simulations are often designed to train teams on how to work together in a real-world setting.
- **Identification and improvement of hazards**: In-situ simulation can be used to identify and improve hazards in the patient care environment. For example, an in-situ simulation can be used to test the response plan for a cardiac arrest event.

Disadvantages of In-Situ Simulation

- **Disruption to patient care**: In-situ simulation may disrupt patient care when not meticulously planned and executed, as it often necessitates the utilization of patient care areas and equipment.
- **Higher cost**: In-situ simulation can incur greater expenses compared to other simulation methods due to the necessity of specialized equipment and staffing.
- **Complex logistics**: Coordinating in-situ simulation can pose more significant challenges than other simulation types, as it involves multiple departments and staff members.
- **Anxiety and stress in healthcare professionals**: The immersive nature of in-situ simulation can trigger anxiety and stress in healthcare professionals.
- **Risk of injuries**: In some cases, in-situ simulation, especially mock codes, can potentially lead to injuries among healthcare professionals or patients. It is critically important that any simulation medications or equipment is carefully inventoried before and after each simulation to prevent use with actual patients.

Tips for Introducing In-Situ Simulation

- Start by identifying the learning objectives for the in-situ simulation.
- Select a scenario that is relevant to the target audience.
- Coordinate with the hospital leadership, relevant departments, and staff members to ensure that the in-situ simulation does not disrupt patient care.
- Provide training to the staff who will be involved in the in-situ simulation.
- Debrief with the learners after the in-situ simulation to discuss their performance and provide feedback.

By following these tips, you can successfully introduce in situ simulation into your organization.

5.3   Mobile Unit Simulation

Mobile units are simulation centers that are located on vehicles. This allows them to bring healthcare simulation training directly to healthcare facilities. Mobile unit simulation is often used to train healthcare professionals in rural or underserved areas (Baily, 2022).

Mobile units typically have a variety of simulation rooms that are equipped with high-technology mannequins, task trainers, and other equipment. They also have experienced staff who can facilitate simulations and provide feedback to learners.

Examples of Mobile Unit Simulation

- During the COVID-19 pandemic, mobile units traveled to numerous hospitals to prepare clinicians from other specialties to work in intensive care through a hands-on "ICU Provider Mobile Bootcamp." (https://www.medstarhealth. org/news-and-publications/news/mi2s-medstar-sitel-mobile-simulation-lab-dep loyed-in-april-2020-for-covid-19-response).
- A team of nurses and physicians can be trained on how to respond to a code blue in a rural hospital with a mobile training unit (Fig. 5.3).
- A new surgeon can be trained on how to perform a complex surgical procedure in a community hospital on mobile unit simulation.

Advantages of Mobile Unit Simulation

- **Space savings**: Mobile unit simulation can free up space inside the healthcare facility because the training is conducted outside.
- **Shared resources**: Expensive simulation and support equipment can be shared across many facilities.
- **Easy access for participants**: Mobile unit simulation is conveniently located just a short walk outdoors for participants. There is no need to plan for transit time to and from a fixed simulation center.

Disadvantages of Mobile Unit Simulation

- **Limited training capacity:** Mobile units typically have a smaller training capacity compared to dedicated simulation centers. This can limit the number of learners who can be trained simultaneously and the frequency with which training can be conducted.
- **Cost-effectiveness**: While mobile units may be more cost-effective than building and maintaining a dedicated simulation center, the overall cost can still be high, especially when factoring in the costs of transportation, setup, and equipment maintenance.

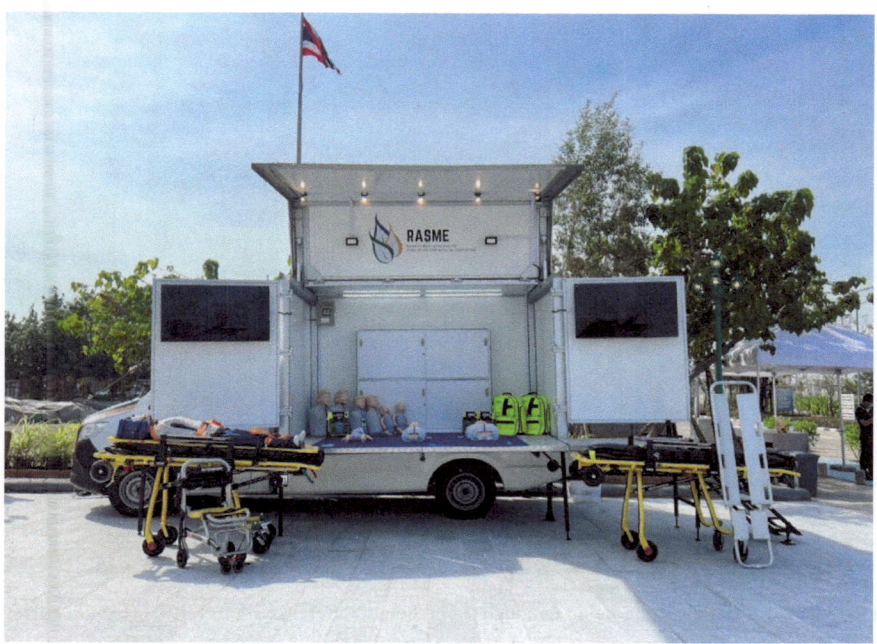

Fig. 5.3 Mobile unit simulation (*photo courtesy* Ramathibodi Academy of Simulation for Medical Education)

5.4 Ad Hoc Simulation (Off-Site)

Ad hoc simulation, also known as off-site simulation, is a type of simulation-based medical education conducted in a non-traditional or makeshift setting. Unlike traditional simulation-based medical education, which typically takes place in dedicated simulation centers with high-technology manikins and specialized equipment, ad hoc simulation utilizes readily available resources and equipment in a variety of settings.

Ad hoc simulation is often used to train healthcare professionals in specific clinical settings or teams working in different locations. It can also be used to train on specific equipment or procedures that may not be available in a dedicated simulation center.

Examples of Ad Hoc Simulation

- Bringing simulation equipment to a convention center to conduct difficult airway simulations at an emergency medicine conference.
- Converting hotel rooms or conference rooms into simulation rooms to allow for conducting simulations for competency assessment (Fig. 5.4).

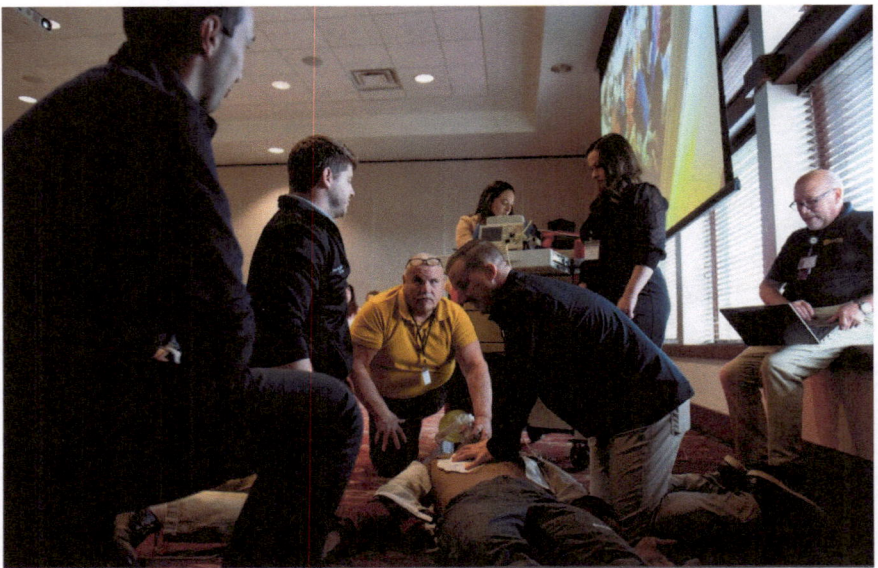

Fig. 5.4 Ad hoc simulation being conducted in a hotel conference room setting (*photo courtesy* WISER)

Advantages of Ad Hoc Simulation

- **Accessibility**: Ad hoc simulation can bring training directly to learners, reducing the need for travel. This approach brings the capabilities of a simulation center to a setting outside the confines of a simulation center or healthcare facility.

Disadvantages of Ad Hoc Simulation

- **Logistics coordination**: Coordinating the logistics of ad hoc simulation can be challenging. The equipment must be transported to the off-site facility including supporting equipment
- **Resource limitations**: Ad hoc simulation may be limited by the available resources at the off-site location. Examples include difficulty with Wi-Fi and other technology access points that are taken for granted inside of simulation centers.
- **Non-Customized Facilities**: The facilities used for ad hoc simulations lack custom designs to accommodate the wide range of equipment utilized for simulation. This includes challenges related to hanging overhead equipment, establishing cable pathways and tracks, and ensuring control over lighting and sound equipment.

5.5 Summary

The choice of simulation setting depends on a number of factors, including the learning objectives, the target audience, the available resources, and the potential benefits and drawbacks of each setting. Examples of different settings include in traditional simulation centers, in-situ simulation in healthcare settings, mobile unit simulation and ad hoc settings.

Traditional simulation centers offer a safe and controlled environment for simulation-based education with access to specialized equipment and experienced staff. However, simulation centers can be expensive to build and maintain and may not be accessible to all healthcare professionals.

In-situ simulation is a valuable tool for training healthcare professionals in a realistic and engaging environment. However, in-situ simulation can be disruptive to patient care and can be more expensive and difficult to coordinate than other types of simulation.

Mobile unit simulation allows us to train healthcare professionals in rural or underserved areas. However, the mobile unit simulation setting might not be as well-equipped as a traditional simulation center or an in-situ simulation space.

Ad hoc (off-site) simulation allows the simulation to occur in a non-traditional environment. This type of simulation can support a group of healthcare providers or students without access to a simulation center or to medical institution supporting in situ simulation.

References

Anderson, E. R., Black, R., & Brocklehurst, P. (2005). Acute obstetric emergency drill in England and Wales: A survey of practice. *BJOG: an International Journal of Obstetrics & Gynaecology, 112*(3), 372–375. https://doi.org/10.1111/j.1471-0528.2005.00432.x

Baily, L. (2022, July 21). Mobile simulation centers help train learners on the go. HealthySimulation.com. Accessed October 31, 2023. https://www.healthysimulation.com/44065/mobile-simulation-center-benefits/

MI2s MedStar SiTEL Mobile Simulation Lab deployed in April 2020 for COVID-19 response. Accessed October 31, 2023. https://www.medstarhealth.org/news-and-publications/news/mi2s-medstar-sitel-mobile-simulation-lab-deployed-in-april-2020-for-covid-19-response

Phrampus, P. E. (2014, June 20). Insitu mock codes evaluate people readiness and system readiness—An important patient safety tool. *Simulating Healthcare.* A blog dedicated to discussions and relevant things regarding simulation in healthcare. Accessed October 23, 2023. https://simulatinghealthcare.net/2014/06/20/insitu-mock-codes-evaluate-people-readiness-and-system-readiness-an-important-patient-safety-tool/

Sørensen, J. L., Lottrup, P., van der Vleuten, C., et al. (2014). Unannounced in situ simulation of obstetric emergencies: Staff perceptions and organisational impact. *Postgraduate Medical Journal, 90*(1069), 622–629. https://doi.org/10.1136/postgradmedj-2013-132280

Sørensen, J. L., Østergaard, D., LeBlanc, V., et al. (2017). Design of simulation-based medical education and advantages and disadvantages of in situ simulation versus off-site simulation. *BMC Medical Education, 17*, 20. https://doi.org/10.1186/s12909-016-0838-3

Chapter 6
Scenario Design

Abstract The process of designing effective healthcare simulation scenarios involves four key steps to ensure focused, well-organized, and goal-aligned educational experiences. Firstly, selecting a topic that addresses learners' needs and aligns with program goals is paramount. This requires considering available resources, engaging topics, and appropriateness for learners' experience levels. Secondly, identifying the target learner group based on their experience, qualifications, learning preferences, and cultural backgrounds is crucial for tailoring scenarios to their needs. Thirdly, clearly defining learning objectives that are SMART (Specific, Measurable, Achievable, Relevant, and Time-bound) provides a roadmap for focused scenario design. Lastly, developing a comprehensive assessment plan, including learning objectives, assessment criteria, tools, and feedback strategies, ensures the evaluation aligns with educational goals and supports ongoing program improvement. Additionally, the creation of a simulation story involves crafting a compelling narrative with three key phases—stem, information offered, and information elicited—guiding learners through immersive scenarios. Considerations such as fidelity, realism, debriefing, and regular scenario evaluation contribute to designing impactful simulation scenarios that enhance healthcare professionals' learning and development, ultimately improving patient care outcomes.

Keywords Topic · Learner · Learning objectives · Assessment plan · Simulation story · Scenario design

A simulation scenario is an artificial representation of a real-world event to achieve educational goals through experiential learning. Designing an effective simulation scenario requires careful planning and can be broken into several steps. A structured approach to scenario design can help ensure that simulations are focused, well-organized, and aligned with specific learning objectives (Harrington & Simon, 2023 Miller et al., 2021; O'Donnell & Phrampus, 2017; Phrampus, 2018; Watts et al., 2021). Here are the first four steps to guide the crafting of effective healthcare simulation scenarios (O'Donnell & Phrampus, 2017; Phrampus, 2018) (Fig. 6.1).

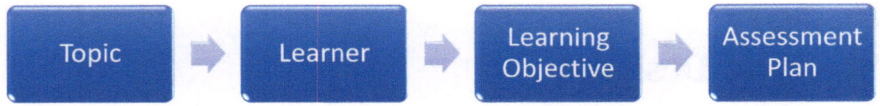

Fig. 6.1 The four critical steps in simulation scenario design

6.1   Step 1: Select a Topic

The first step involves choosing a topic that aligns with the learners' needs and the overall goals of the simulation training curriculum. This topic should be relevant to the learners' level of experience and expertise. For instance, a simulation for advanced practice nurses might focus on managing complex patient cases of chest pain, while a simulation for newly graduated nurses might focus on basic nursing skills and procedures.

Here are some tips for selecting a topic for a simulation scenario:

- Start with the learners' needs. What do the learners need to learn in order to meet their professional goals?
- Consider the overall goals of the training program. What are the specific skills or knowledge that the training program is trying to impart?
- Be realistic about the available resources. What resources are available to support the simulation?
- Choose a topic that is engaging and relevant to the learners. The learners are more likely to be motivated to learn if the topic is interesting to them.
- Make sure that the topic is appropriate for the level of experience of the learners. The simulation scenario should not be too easy or too difficult for the learners.

6.2   Step 2: Define the Learners

Identifying the target learner group is crucial for tailoring the simulation scenario to their specific needs and capabilities. Consider the learners' level of training, experience, and prior knowledge. This will help determine the complexity of the scenario and the depth of information to be covered.

Here are some aspects to consider when identifying learners for a simulation-based educational session:

1. **Experience Level**: Determine the learners' level of experience in the clinical area being simulated. For example, a simulation for advanced practice nurses may require more experience than a simulation for newly graduated nurses.
2. **Professional Background**: Identify the learners' professional background and qualifications. This can help determine the depth of knowledge and skills that can be assumed.

3. **Learning Preferences**: Determine the learners' preferred learning styles and adapt the simulation scenario accordingly. Some learners may prefer a more hands-on approach, while others may benefit from a more theoretical approach.
4. **Cultural Background**: Consider the learners' cultural background and adapt the scenario to avoid any unintended biases or misunderstandings. This ensures that the scenario is inclusive and respectful of all participants.

Benefits of Effective Learner Identification

- **Enhances Learning Outcomes**: Tailoring the simulation scenario to the learners' needs and capabilities helps them achieve the desired learning outcomes.
- **Learning Objectives**: Identifying the learners will help to inform the specifics of developing the learning objectives.
- **Promotes Engagement**: Learners are more likely to be engaged and motivated if the scenario is relevant to their level of experience and learning goals.
- **Creates a Safe Learning Environment**: By understanding the learners' skill level, instructors can minimize the risk of frustration or anxiety during the simulation.
- **Optimizes Resource Allocation**: Tailoring the scenario to the learners' needs helps instructors allocate resources efficiently and effectively.

Strategies for Learner Identification

- **Review of Learner Profiles**: Accessing records or profiles of the learners can provide insights into their experience, qualifications, and learning preferences.
- **Pre-Simulation Assessments**: Conducting pre-simulation assessments can help gauge the learners' knowledge and skills in the specific clinical area being simulated.
- **Learner Self-Assessment**: Asking learners to complete a self-assessment questionnaire can provide information about their experience, learning goals, and preferred learning styles.
- **Communication with Instructors or Supervisors**: Communicating with instructors or supervisors who have worked with the learners can provide valuable insights into their strengths, weaknesses, and learning preferences.

6.3 Step 3: Design the Learning Objectives

Learning objectives are clearly defined statements that describe what learners should be able to know or do as a result of participating in a learning activity or experience. They provide clarity and direction for both instructors and learners, ensuring that the learning experience is focused and aligned with specific goals.

Characteristics of Effective Learning Objectives are SMART (Specific, Measurable, Attainable, Relevant, and Time-bound) (Doran, 1981). They should be:

- **Specific**: Clearly defined and focused on a specific skill, knowledge, or behavior.

- **Measurable**: Able to be assessed or evaluated to determine whether the objective has been achieved.
- **Attainable**: Realistic and aligned with the learners' level of experience and the available resources.
- **Relevant**: Connected to the overall goals of the learning activity or experience.
- **Time-bound**: Specify a timeframe for achieving the objective.

Examples of Learning Objectives in Healthcare Simulation

- **Cardiopulmonary resuscitation (CPR)**: Upon completion of the 10 min scenario, learners will be able to:

    – Demonstrate the correct hand placement and compression depth for CPR
    – Effectively ventilate a patient using bag-valve-mask ventilation
    – Identify and manage common complications during CPR

- **Intubation and ventilation**: Upon completion of the scenario, learners will be able to:

    – Properly prepare and administer anesthesia for intubation within 5 min
    – Successfully intubate a patient using the correct technique
    – Manage potential complications during and after intubation

- **Trauma management**: Upon completion of the scenario, learners will be able to:

    – Conduct a primary trauma survey and identify critical injuries within 2 min
    – Prioritize treatment based on the patient's injuries
    – Effectively stabilize the patient for transport

- **Critical care**: Upon completion of the 15 min scenario, learners will be able to:

    – Monitor and interpret critical patient data
    – Recognize and respond to early signs of deterioration
    – Apply appropriate critical care interventions to stabilize the patient.

Learning objectives serve as a roadmap for designing effective simulation scenarios and evaluating learner performance. They ensure that the simulation experience is purposeful, focused, and aligned with the desired learning outcomes. Overall, learning objectives are essential elements in simulation-based education, providing both instructors and learners with clear direction and a framework for assessing the effectiveness of the learning experience.

6.4   Step 4: Develop the Assessment Plan

An assessment plan determines how the learners' performance will be evaluated against the established learning objectives. This plan may involve checklists, rating scales, or other assessment tools. Or in some cases it may be as simple as the faculty members giving feedback to the leaners based on professional judgement. The assessment plan should be designed to provide constructive feedback and guide learners in their areas for improvement.

Components of an Assessment Plan

- **Learning Objectives**: Clearly defined learning objectives serve as the foundation for the assessment plan. They specify what learners are expected to know or do as a result of participating in the simulation.
- **Assessment Criteria**: Based on the learning objectives, assessment criteria are developed to identify the specific skills, knowledge, and behaviors that will be evaluated. These criteria should be aligned with the learning objectives and be observable and measurable.
- **Assessment Tools**: Depending on the nature of the learning objectives and assessment criteria, appropriate assessment tools are selected. These tools may include checklists, rating scales, rubrics, or written reports.
- **Feedback Strategy**: A well-structured feedback strategy is essential for providing learners with constructive and actionable feedback. Feedback should be specific, timely, and focused on helping learners improve their performance.
- **Evaluation of the Assessment Plan**: It is important to regularly evaluate the effectiveness of the assessment plan and make adjustments as needed. This ensures that the assessment plan remains relevant, accurate, and aligned with the learning objectives.

Benefits of Effective Assessment Plans

- **Enhanced Learning**: Learners benefit from clear expectations and receive valuable feedback that can guide their learning process.
- **Improved Performance**: Instructors can identify areas where learners need additional support and provide targeted interventions to improve their performance.
- **Program Evaluation**: Assessment data can be used to evaluate the overall effectiveness of the simulation-based medical education program and identify areas for improvement.
- **Enhanced Professionalism**: The assessment process helps learners develop self-reflection and evaluation skills, essential for professional development.

In conclusion, assessment plans are integral components of effective simulation-based medical education programs. They provide a structured approach to evaluating learners' performance, facilitate meaningful feedback, and contribute to ongoing program improvement. By developing and implementing appropriate assessment plans instructors can foster a high-quality learning environment that maximizes the benefits of simulation-based medical education.

6.5   Crafting the Simulation Story

Once the four core steps are completed, the next stage involves developing the actual simulation story. This is where the scenario is brought to life by incorporating details, character development, and a logical progression of events that allow an assessment of the learners to occur upon completion of the activity. The story should engage the learners and guide them through the scenario in a way that fosters the desired learning outcomes (O'Donnell & Phrampus, 2017).

The story is typically divided into three sections.

1. **Stem**: The Stem serves as the opening hook, a concise and captivating statement that immediately immerses the learners in the scenario, piquing their curiosity and setting the stage for the unfolding events.
2. **Information Offered**: The second phase presents readily available information to the learners, mimicking the data they would access in a real-world clinical setting. This information could be found on patient charts, through handoffs from other healthcare providers, or through passive observation. Information should be limited to that which is important to accomplishing the learning objectives.
3. **Information Elicited**: The third phase challenges the learners to actively gather essential information, simulating the process of clinical assessment and questioning. This information is not explicitly provided but must be unearthed through astute questioning, critical observation, and clinical reasoning.

Example of the Three Phases of Story Development

Stem: A 25-year-old female with a history of asthma presents to the emergency department with difficulty breathing. She reports that her symptoms started approximately two hours ago and have been worsening despite using her albuterol inhaler at home. She is currently using accessory muscles to breathe and is experiencing wheezing and shortness of breath.

Information Offered

- Vital signs: Blood pressure 120/80 mmHg, heart rate 130 beats per minute, respiratory rate 30 breaths per minute, temperature 37.0 °C
- Past medical history: Asthma diagnosed at age 5, no hospitalizations for asthma in the past year
- Social history: No smoking, no alcohol or drug use
- Medication history: Albuterol inhaler as needed
- Allergies: No known allergies.

Information Elicited

- Physical exam: Alert and oriented, using accessory muscles to breathe, wheezing on inspiration and expiration, lungs hyperinflated
- Oxygen saturation: 88% on room air

- After the patient was given bronchodilator, the symptoms relieve

In addition to the steps of scenario design above, here are some additional considerations for effective scenario design:

1. **Fidelity**: Determine the appropriate level of fidelity for the simulation, considering the learning objectives and available resources. High-technology manikins and specialized equipment may be appropriate for complex scenarios, while low-technology mannequins and task trainers may suffice for basic skill development.
2. **Realism**: Strive to create a realistic environment that mimics the actual clinical setting where the skills or procedures being practiced are typically performed. This enhances the immersion experience and reinforces the transferability of the learned skills to real-world practice. The environment should be free of distracting elements that are not required to accomplish the learning objectives.
3. **Debriefing**: Plan for a well-structured debriefing session following the simulation. This is where learners reflect on their experiences, receive feedback, and discuss strategies for improvement. The debriefing should be facilitated by an experienced instructor who can guide the learners through the learning process.
4. **Evaluation and Refinement**: Evaluate the effectiveness of the simulation scenario after its implementation. Gather feedback from learners, facilitators, and other stakeholders to identify areas for improvement. Regularly refine the scenario based on this feedback to ensure it remains relevant, effective, and aligned with the learning objectives.

By following these steps and considering the additional factors mentioned, healthcare professionals can design effective simulation scenarios that enhance the learning and development of their colleagues, ultimately improving patient care outcomes.

References

Doran, G. T. (1981). There's a SMART way to write management's goals and objectives. *Management Review, 70*(11), 35–36.

Harrington, D. W., & Simon, L. V. (2023). Designing a simulation scenario. In: *StatPearls*. StatPearls Publishing. Accessed November 22, 2023. http://www.ncbi.nlm.nih.gov/books/NBK547670/

Miller, C., Deckers, C., Jones, M., Wells-Beede, E., & McGee, E. (2021). Healthcare Simulation Standards of Best Practice™ outcomes and objectives. *Clinical Simulation in Nursing, 58*, 40–44. https://doi.org/10.1016/j.ecns.2021.08.013

O'Donnell, J., & Phrampus, P. (2017). Simulation in nurse anesthesia. In: B. Henrich & J. Thompson (Eds.), *A resource for nurse anesthesia educators* (5th ed., pp. 261–294). American Association of Nurse Anesthetists.

Phrampus, P. E. (2018, July 23). The first four steps of healthcare simulation scenario design. *Simulating Healthcare*. A blog dedicated to discussions and relevant things regarding simulation in healthcare. Accessed November 22, 2023. https://simulatinghealthcare.net/2018/07/23/the-first-four-steps-of-healthcare-simulation-scenario-design/

Watts, P. I., McDermott, D. S., Alinier, G., et al. (2021). Healthcare Simulation Standards of Best Practice™ simulation design. *Clinical Simulation in Nursing, 58*, 14–21. https://doi.org/10.1016/j.ecns.2021.08.009

Chapter 7
Simulation Phases

Abstract Simulation-based education (SBE) incorporates five essential phases to create an effective and immersive learning experience for healthcare professionals. These phases, detailed in the comprehensive discussion, are preparation, briefing, simulation activity, debriefing, and application. The preparation phase involves setting the stage by providing an overview of the scenario, addressing concerns, and introducing relevant concepts. Briefing formalizes expectations and clarifies roles, safety protocols, and logistics. The simulation activity, the core phase, immerses learners in realistic scenarios, allowing them to apply knowledge and skills in a controlled environment. Debriefing is a critical phase where learners reflect, receive feedback, and identify areas for improvement. Lastly, the application phase focuses on transferring learned skills and knowledge to real-world practice, contributing to improved patient care outcomes. Effective implementation of these phases maximizes skill development and prepares healthcare professionals for the complexities of clinical practice. References provided support the evidence-based practices in SBME, emphasizing the importance of each phase in achieving desired educational outcomes.

Based on a review of research on skill acquisition, Ericsson identified a set of conditions where practice had been uniformly associated with improved performance. Significant performance improvements were realized when individuals were (1) given a task with a well-defined goal, (2) motivated to improve, (3) provided with feedback, and (4) provided with ample opportunities for repetition and gradual refinements of their performance (Anders, 2008) By incorporating these principles into the five phases of simulation-based medical education—preparation, briefing, simulation activity, debriefing, and application—learners can maximize their learning from simulations and significantly improve their clinical skills and decision-making abilities (Fig. 7.1).

Fig. 7.1 Phases of
simulation

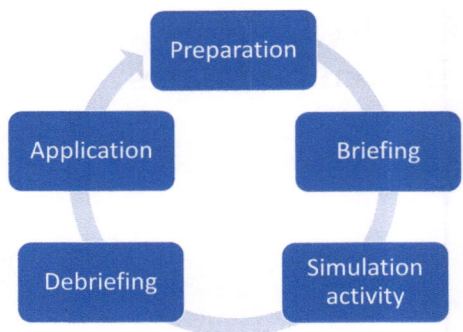

7.1   Preparation: Setting the Stage for Learning

Before embarking on the simulation experience, preparing the learners by providing an overview of the upcoming scenario is crucial. The preparation phase may be called pre-briefing or pre-course phase. This establishes expectations, addresses any questions or concerns, and introduces relevant concepts or skills (McDermott et al., 2021; Phrampus, 2021).

Objectives of the Preparation Phase

- **Establish expectations**: Clearly define the simulation's purpose, the learners' roles and responsibilities, and the desired learning outcomes.
- **Provide background information**: Share relevant background information, research findings, or theoretical concepts related to the simulation topic.
- **Assign pre-reading or assignments**: If necessary, assign pre-reading materials or exercises to familiarize learners with the topic or skills being addressed.
- **Address learner concerns**: Answer any questions or address any concerns that learners may have about the simulation experience.

Elements of the Preparation Phase

- **Articulation of learning objectives**: Clearly define the specific learning objectives the learners are expected to achieve through the simulation experience. Depending on the design of the simulation, this may be deferred to the debriefing if it is necessary to preserve a diagnostic mystery during the case.
- **Discussion of relevant background information**: Share any relevant background information, research findings, or theoretical concepts to enhance the learning experience.
- **Assignment of pre-reading or exercises**: If necessary, assign pre-reading materials or exercises to familiarize learners with the topic or skills being addressed.
- **Overview of the simulation course or scenario**: Provide a general outline of the simulation content, including the patient presentation, setting, potential complications, and the expected simulation duration.

- **Introduction of simulation methodologies**: If learners are new to simulation, provide an overview of the simulation methodologies used, such as high-technology manikins or standardized patients.
- **Introduction to the Simulated Environment**: The learner(s) should be oriented to the environment of the simulation with particular attention to the equipment available, location of data sources (if any: Vital Signs for example) as well as anything else that is relevant to their decision making during the scenario.

At the Winter Institute for Simulation, Education and Research (WISER), most of the preparation phase elements are incorporated into our online platform, the WISER Simulation Information Management System (SIMS™). This affords learners the opportunity to be better prepared to engage in the planned simulation activity.

Strategies for Effective Preparation Phase

- **Tailor the material to the learners' needs and knowledge level**: Adapt the content to the learners' specific needs and knowledge level.
- **Engage learners actively**: Use interactive methods such as discussions, polls, or case studies to engage learners in the pre-briefing process actively.
- **Create a welcoming and supportive learning environment**: Foster a safe and supportive environment where learners feel comfortable asking questions and sharing their thoughts.
- **Emphasize the relevance of simulation to clinical practice**: Highlight the connection between the simulation experience and real-world clinical practice to enhance motivation and engagement.

By carefully planning and implementing the preparation phase, instructors can prepare learners for a meaningful and successful simulation experience. This initial step lays the foundation for effective learning. It ensures that learners are well-equipped to engage in the simulation activity and clearly understand the objectives and expectations.

7.2 Briefing: Establishing the Rules of Engagement

Immediately before the simulation activity, a formal briefing sets the stage for the learners' participation. It is a structured orientation session that sets the stage for learners' participation, outlining the roles, responsibilities, safety protocols, and expectations for the upcoming scenario.

Purpose of the Briefing

- **Establish Role Clarity**: Clearly define the roles and responsibilities of each learner, ensuring they understand their assigned tasks and actions within the simulation scenario (Hughes & Hughes, 2023; McDermott et al., 2021; Phrampus, 2020).

- **Set Expectations**: Establish clear expectations regarding the simulation objectives, timeline, and anticipated events, aligning learners' understanding with the instructor's vision for the scenario. Ensure the learners are clear on the intended rule of engagement regarding student/student interactions during the scenario which may range from none, to considerable depending on the scenario design.
- **Review Safety Protocols**: Reinforce safety protocols and ethical considerations, emphasizing communication channels, emergency procedures, and boundaries for learner interactions.
- **Manage Logistics**: Address any logistical aspects, such as the location of the simulation equipment, necessary resources, and technical arrangements.
- **Address Learner Questions**: Facilitate an open discussion, allowing learners to ask questions, clarify any concerns, and gain a comprehensive understanding of the simulation scenario.

Content of the Briefing

- **Scenario Overview**: Provide a brief overview of the simulation scenario, including the patient presentation, setting, potential complications, and the expected duration of the simulation.
- **Role Assignment**: Assign roles to each learner, ensuring they understand their responsibilities and actions within the simulation.
- **Safety Protocols**: Reiterate safety protocols, emphasizing communication channels, emergency procedures, and ethical considerations.
- **Fidelity Expectations**: Clarify the level of fidelity, such as high-technology manikins or low-technology task trainers, to manage expectations.
- **Learning Objectives**: Reiterate the specific learning objectives the learners are expected to achieve through the simulation experience.

Strategies for Effective Briefing

- **Concise and Focused**: Keep the briefing concise and focused, providing only essential information to avoid overwhelming learners.
- **Interactive Engagement**: Use interactive methods, such as role-playing scenarios or Q&A sessions, to actively engage learners and enhance their understanding.
- **Tailored to Learner Needs**: Adapt the briefing to the learners' needs and knowledge level, ensuring the information is relevant and applicable to their experience.
- **Open Communication**: Foster an open communication environment where learners feel comfortable asking questions and seeking clarification.
- **Realistic Expectations**: Set realistic expectations for the simulation, ensuring that learners understand the level of challenge and the learning opportunities it presents.

By conducting a well-structured and informative briefing, instructors can prepare learners for a meaningful and successful simulation experience. This briefing sets the stage for effective engagement, ensures learners are well-equipped to fulfill their assigned roles, and fosters a safe and supportive learning environment.

7.3 Simulation Activity: The Immersive Learning Experience

In simulation-based medical education, the simulation activity serves as the core component of the learning experience. During this immersive and interactive phase, learners engage with the meticulously crafted scenario, applying their knowledge, skills, and decision-making abilities in a safe and controlled environment. The simulation activity encompasses the actual execution of the scenario, where learners interact with simulated patients, manikins, or standardized patients, mimicking real-world clinical encounters (Persico et al., 2021).

Objectives of the Simulation Activity

- **Provide a safe and realistic environment**: Create a safe environment that replicates real-world clinical practice's challenges and complexities at a level that enable the accomplishment of the learning objectives, allowing learners to train their skills and decision-making abilities without compromising patient safety.
- **Enhance skill development**: Foster the development of clinical skills, procedural techniques, and communication competencies through hands-on practice and exposure to diverse patient presentations.
- **Promote critical thinking and problem-solving**: Encourage critical thinking and problem-solving skills as learners analyze patient data, identify potential complications, and formulate effective treatment plans.
- **Facilitate collaboration and teamwork**: Enhance teamwork and collaboration skills as learners work together to assess, manage, and care for simulated patients.

Key Elements of the Simulation Activity

- **Appropriate simulation environment**: Use modalities, such as manikins, standardized patients, or virtual reality tools, to create an environment that allows the accomplishment of the learning objectives.
- **Scenario progression**: Guide the scenario progression through carefully designed scripts, introducing unexpected events, complications, and patient deterioration to challenge learners' decision-making abilities **and allow them to accomplish the learning objectives**.
- **Facilitator monitoring**: Maintain ongoing monitoring of the simulation activity by a well-prepared facilitator, providing cues or prompts when necessary to accomplish the learning objectives.
- **Technical support**: Ensure seamless environmental set up, operation of simulation equipment and technology to avoid disruptions to the learning experience.

Strategies for Effective Simulation Activity

- **Align scenario with learning objectives**: Tailor the simulation scenario to align with the specific learning objectives for the target learner group.

- **Incorporate realistic patient presentations**: Design patient presentations that reflect the diversity of clinical encounters, including varied ages, backgrounds, and medical conditions necessary to accomplish the learning objectives.
- **Encourage active learner engagement**: Promote active learner engagement by encouraging participation, questioning, and collaborative decision-making within the simulation.

By carefully designing and implementing the simulation activity, instructors can create a stimulating and challenging learning environment that allows learners to apply their knowledge, skills, and decision-making abilities in a safe setting. This immersive experience fosters the development of essential clinical competencies and prepares learners for the complexities of real-world healthcare practice.

7.4   Debriefing: Extracting Meaningful Learning

The debriefing session is a crucial component of simulation-based medical education, allowing learners to reflect on their experiences, receive feedback, and identify areas for improvement. The debriefing should be facilitated by an experienced instructor who can guide the learners through the learning process (Decker et al., 2021; Phrampus & O'Donnell, 2013). The debriefing typically includes:

- **Reflection and Sharing**: Encourage learners to share their perspectives, emotions, and actions during the simulation.
- **Feedback and Analysis**: Provide constructive feedback on individual and group performance, highlighting strengths and areas for improvement.
- **Open Discussion**: Facilitate an open discussion, allowing learners to ask questions, address concerns, and engage in peer-to-peer learning.
- **Objective Identification**: Help learners identify specific learning objectives that were achieved and those that require further attention.

We will intensely discuss debriefing in the following two chapters.

7.5   Application: Transferring Learning to Practice

The ultimate goal of simulation-based medical education is to facilitate the transfer of learned skills and knowledge to real-world practice. The application phase of simulation-based medical education goes beyond individual learner performance. It focuses on the real-world impact of simulation-based medical education on patient care and public health outcomes (McGaghie et al., 2010, 2011; Paganotti & Chidume, 2023). This phase aligns seamlessly with the three levels of translational science in health professions education:

- **T1 Level: From Simulation Laboratory to Learning Outcomes**

This level focuses on designing and delivering educational protocols within the controlled environment of the simulation laboratory. The primary focus is measuring educational outcomes, such as knowledge acquisition, skill development, and learner confidence. Many existing simulation-based medical education studies fall within this level, evaluating the effectiveness of specific simulation interventions in improving learner performance.

- **T2 Level: Bridging the Gap to Patient Care Delivery**

This second level extends the application of simulation-based medical education findings beyond the laboratory setting. The goal is to translate the acquired knowledge and skills into better patient care delivery practices, such as implementing ACLS protocols or managing complicated obstetric deliveries. This level focuses on measuring the impact of simulation-based medical education on specific clinical processes and procedures, demonstrating the link between improved learner performance and enhanced patient care.

- **T3 Level: Linking Simulation Education to Patient Outcomes**

This level represents the third goal of translational science in simulation-based medical education, where the focus shifts to improved patient outcomes. This involves measuring the direct impact of educational interventions, such as skillful laparoscopic surgery, on measurable outcomes like faster patient recovery as a result of improved healthcare practices.

- **T4 Level: Linking Simulation Education to Population Outcomes, Finances or Regulatory Change**

This fourth level represents the final stage of translation science applied to simulation. Outcomes such as improved infection rates, reduced insurance premiums, changes to regulatory requirements or calculation of return on investment for simulation fall into this category.

Strategies for Effective Application

- **Provide ongoing support**: Offer ongoing support and mentoring to learners as they apply their simulation learnings to their clinical practice.
- **Promote reflective practice**: Encourage reflective practice by prompting learners to analyze their clinical experiences and identify opportunities for improvement.
- **Facilitate peer-to-peer learning**: Foster peer-to-peer learning by creating opportunities for learners to share their experiences, insights, and best practices with colleagues.
- **Integrate simulation into training programs**: Incorporate simulation based educational methodologies and debriefing techniques into ongoing training programs and clinical rotations.

- **Measure and evaluate outcomes**: Develop metrics to evaluate the impact of simulation based education on learner performance, patient outcomes, and healthcare quality.

By integrating these insights, the application phase of simulation-based medical education can evolve beyond individual learner performance and contribute to the advancement of knowledge and health care delivery. By focusing on T2 and T3 level outcomes, we can ensure that our simulation-based medical education efforts have a lasting and positive impact on the lives of patients and communities.

7.6 Summary

Simulation-based medical education utilizes five phases to create a safe and immersive learning environment for healthcare professionals. These phases work together to maximize skill development and prepare learners for real-world clinical practice.

1. **Preparation**: This sets the stage by providing background information, outlining objectives, and addressing any concerns. The goal is to ensure learners are well-equipped for the upcoming scenario.
2. **Briefing**: This formalizes expectations and clarifies roles for each learner. It establishes safety protocols, logistics, and the scenario's rules of engagement. A clear and concise briefing ensures everyone is on the same page.
3. **Simulation Activity**: This core phase places learners in the heart of the scenario, where they apply their knowledge and skills in a realistic setting. Scenarios can involve manikins, standardized patients, or virtual reality tools. Instructors monitor and guide the activity to ensure objectives are met.
4. **Debriefing**: This crucial phase helps learners reflect on their experiences, receive constructive feedback, and identify areas for improvement. An open and facilitated discussion allows for peer-to-peer learning and solidifies the key takeaways from the simulation.
5. **Application**: This final phase focuses on transferring learning to real-world practice. It goes beyond individual performance and examines the impact of simulation-based medical education on patient care and public health outcomes. Effective application involves ongoing support, reflective practice, and integration of simulation-based medical education methodologies into clinical training.

By effectively implementing these five phases, simulation-based medical education can significantly improve clinical skills, decision-making abilities, and ultimately, patient care.

References

Anders, E. K. (2008). Deliberate practice and acquisition of expert performance: A general overview. *Academic Emergency Medicine, 15*(11), 988–994. https://doi.org/10.1111/j.1553-2712.2008.00227.x

Decker, S., Alinier, G., Crawford, S. B., Gordon, R. M., Jenkins, D., & Wilson, C. (2021). Healthcare Simulation Standards of Best Practice™ the debriefing process. *Clinical Simulation in Nursing, 58*, 27–32. https://doi.org/10.1016/j.ecns.2021.08.011

Hughes, P. G., & Hughes, K. E. (2023). Briefing prior to simulation activity. In: *StatPearls*. StatPearls Publishing. Accessed December 6, 2023. http://www.ncbi.nlm.nih.gov/books/NBK545234/

McDermott, D. S., Ludlow, J., Horsley, E., & Meakim, C. (2021). Healthcare Simulation Standards of Best Practice™ prebriefing: Preparation and briefing. *Clinical Simulation in Nursing, 58*, 9–13. https://doi.org/10.1016/j.ecns.2021.08.008

McGaghie, W. C., Draycott, T. J., Dunn, W. F., Lopez, C. M., & Stefanidis, D. (2011). Evaluating the impact of simulation on translational patient outcomes. *Simulation in Healthcare, 6*(7), S42–S47. https://doi.org/10.1097/SIH.0b013e318222fde9

McGaghie, W. C., Issenberg, S. B., Petrusa, E. R., & Scalese, R. J. (2010). A critical review of simulation-based medical education research: 2003–2009. *Medical Education, 44*(1), 50–63. https://doi.org/10.1111/j.1365-2923.2009.03547.x

Pagancti, L., & Chidume, T. (2023). Translational science in medical simulation. In: *StatPearls*. StatPearls Publishing. Accessed December 6, 2023. http://www.ncbi.nlm.nih.gov/books/NBK560752/

Persico, L., Belle, A., DiGregorio, H., Wilson-Keates, B., & Shelton, C. (2021). Healthcare Simulation Standards of Best Practice™ facilitation. *Clinical Simulation in Nursing, 58*, 22–26. https://doi.org/10.1016/j.ecns.2021.08.010

Phrampus, P. E., & O'Donnell, J. M. (2013). Debriefing using a structured and supported approach. In: Levine, A. I., DeMaria, S., Schwartz, A. D., & Sim A. J. (Eds.), *The comprehensive textbook of Healthcare simulation* (pp. 73–84). Springer. https://doi.org/10.1007/978-1-4614-5993-4_6

Phrampus, P. E. (2020, May 7). Exploring the elements of orientation and (pre)briefing in simulation based learning design. *Simulating Healthcare*. A blog dedicated to discussions and relevant things regarding simulation in healthcare. Accessed December 4, 2023. https://simulatinghealthcare.net/2020/05/07/exploring-the-elements-of-orientation-and-prebriefing-in-simulation-based-learning-design/

Phrampus, P. E. (2021, September 21). Five tips for creating hybrid curricula for simulation based learning. *Simulating Healthcare*. A blog dedicated to discussions and relevant things regarding simulation in healthcare in healthcare. Accessed December 4, 2023. https://simulatinghealthcare.net/2021/09/21/five-tips-for-creating-hybrid-curricula-for-simulation-based-learning/

Chapter 8
Feedback and Debriefing

Abstract Debriefing and feedback, while distinct in their nature and objectives, play crucial roles in enhancing learning within simulation-based education (SBE). Debriefing primarily focuses on reflective analysis, promoting self-assessment, identification of performance gaps, and consolidation of knowledge and skills through group discussions guided by various models. It usually occurs after a simulation experience, fostering a safe and supportive environment for open communication. In contrast, feedback centers on providing information about specific performance standards, aiming to bridge performance gaps, offer improvement suggestions, and motivate learners. Feedback can be delivered at various points during or after simulations, requiring clear communication and mutual trust between learners and providers. Both debriefing and feedback contribute to lifelong learning, requiring careful design and delivery within a supportive context, ultimately fostering continuous professional development in the healthcare field. The intrinsic feedback inherent in well-designed simulations further enriches the learning experience by guiding learners through the consequences of their actions, emphasizing the collaborative nature of SBME.

Keywords Feedback · Debriefing · Reflective analysis · Performance gaps

Both debriefing and feedback serve crucial roles in promoting learning. Feedback is defined as information transferred between participants, facilitators, simulators, or peers to improve the understanding of concepts or aspects of performance (Lopreiato et al., 2016). Debriefing is defined as one form of feedback. It is an activity to encourage participants' reflective thinking and provide feedback about their performance while various aspects of the completed simulation are discussed (Lopreiato et al., 2016). They are distinct in their nature and objectives. Here's a breakdown of their key differences and connections (Fig. 8.1).

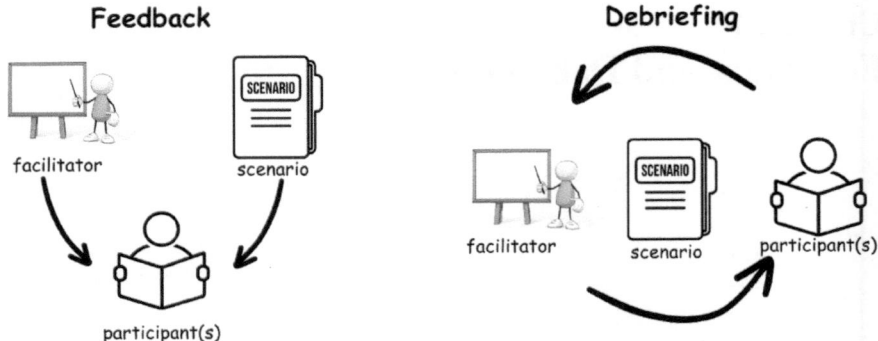

Fig. 8.1 Information flow in feedback and debriefing

8.1   Feedback

Focus: Providing information about the performance of a specific portion of the simulation (Burns, 2015; Voyer & Hatala, 2015).

Objectives:

- Bridge the gap between current performance and desired level.
- Offer suggestions for improvement and future learning.
- Motivate and encourage development.
- Correct actions, or behaviors on the fly during simulations
- Provide direct information to the learner(s) in a simulation.
- Can be used to rescue a simulation (redirecting learners).

Timing: Feedback can occur at various points in the learning process, both during and after the simulation or clinical experience. In some instances, learners may alternate between deliberate practice and receiving directed feedback until they achieve mastery of a skill before moving on to the next set of learning objectives. This specific approach is known as Rapid Cycle Deliberate Practice (RCDP) (Ng et al., 2021).

Structure: This can be formal (e.g., written evaluation) or informal (e.g., verbal coaching) Can be embedded into scenario design as a rescue tool.

Environment: Requires clear communication and mutual trust between the learner and feedback provider.

Role of feedback provider: Deliver feedback in a clear, concise, and timely manner while focusing on specific behaviors and offering actionable suggestions.

Intrinsic Feedback (Phrampus, 2016): Feedback is not always the interaction between students and educators only. Well-designed simulations provide inherent feedback mechanisms that guide learners and offer valuable insights into the consequences of their actions. These intrinsic cues can manifest in various ways:

- **Physiological responses**: Changes in simulated patient vitals, like oxygen saturation improving with supplemental oxygen administration, offer immediate feedback on the effectiveness of interventions.
- **Scenario progression**: The dynamic nature of the scenario itself provides feedback as learners encounter challenges, complications, and unexpected outcomes based on their decisions.
- **Behavioral responses**: Simulated patients may exhibit specific behaviors, verbal cues, emotional responses, or alterations to the script that provide learners with valuable information about the impact of their communication and clinical skills.

By actively participating in these collaborative aspects of the simulation experience, learners gain valuable insights into teamwork dynamics, communication strategies, and collective decision-making, enriching their learning experience.

8.2 Debriefing

Focus: Reflection and analysis of a simulated experience (Burns, 2015; Voyer & Hatala, 2015).

Objectives:

- Promote self-assessment and learning from mistakes as well as correct actions.
- Identify performance gaps and areas for improvement.
- Consolidate knowledge and skills.
- Discuss decisions and rationale.

Timing: This commonly occurs immediately after the simulation experience, usually as a group discussion. Sometimes, the debriefing can occur during a simulation scenario; this technique is called reflective pause, pause and reflect or pause-restart (Clapper, 2010).

Structure: Can be guided by various models; common phases of the debriefing process include reaction/description, understanding/analysis, application/summary (Abulebda et al., 2023).

Environment: Requires a safe and supportive atmosphere for open communication with an understanding that students may experience a sense of vulnerability. The location for debriefing can vary. For example, debriefing can occur in the same environment in which the simulation occurred or be moved to a different location such as a debriefing room. Various learning objectives as well as operational considerations will help to determine the ideal location for the debriefing to occur.

Role of facilitator: Facilitate discussion, guide reflection, and provide constructive feedback while respecting individual perspectives and fostering collaboration. Towards the end of the debriefing help to provide a environment in which there is a summarization of the learned experience of the simulation.

8.3   Connections

- Both debriefing and feedback are tools used to contribute to developing knowledge, skills, and professional judgment.
- Both aim to promote lifelong learning and self-directed improvement.
- Both require careful design and delivery to be effective and meaningful.
- Both are most effective when conducted in a safe and supportive environment that fosters open communication and trust.
- Debriefing can be thought of as a form of feedback that engages the learner in bi-directional information flow that helps the faculty understand the learner's assimilation of the contents of the discussion.

It is important to remember that both debriefing and feedback are essential components of effective learning, and maximizing their impact requires careful consideration of the technical aspects as well as the broader sociocultural and interpersonal contexts. By drawing on insights from simulation and medical education research, educators can continue refining their debriefing and feedback practices, fostering a culture of continuous learning and professional development within the healthcare field.

References

Abulebda, K., Auerbach, M., & Limaiem, F. (2023). Debriefing techniques utilized in medical simulation. In: *StatPearls*. StatPearls Publishing. Accessed December 15, 2023. http://www.ncbi.nlm.nih.gov/books/NBK546660/

Burns, C. L. (2015). Using debriefing and feedback in simulation to improve participant performance: An educator's perspective. *International Journal of Medical Education, 6*, 118–120. https://doi.org/10.5116/ijme.55fb.3d3a

Clapper, T. C. (2010). Beyond Knowles: What those conducting simulation need to know about adult learning theory. *Clinical Simulation in Nursing, 6*(1), e7–e14. https://doi.org/10.1016/j.ecns.2009.07.003

Lopreiato, J. O., Downing, D., Gammon, W., et al. (2016). *Healthcare simulation dictionary*. http://www.ssih.org/dictionary

Ng, C., Primiani, N., & Orchanian-Cheff, A. (2021). Rapid cycle deliberate practice in healthcare simulation: A scoping review. *Medical Science Educator, 31*(6), 2105–2120. https://doi.org/10.1007/s40670-021-01446-0

Phrampus, P. E. (2016, April 25). Learning from simulation—Far more than the debriefing. *Simulating Healthcare*. A blog dedicated to discussions and relevant things regarding simulation in healthcare in healthcare. Accessed December 11, 2023. https://simulatinghealthcare.net/2016/04/25/learning-from-simulation-far-more-than-the-debriefing/

Voyer, S., & Hatala, R. (2015). Debriefing and feedback: Two sides of the same coin? *Simulation in Healthcare, 10*(2), 67. https://doi.org/10.1097/SIH.0000000000000075

Chapter 9
Debriefing

Abstract Debriefing is a pivotal element in simulation-based medical education, serving as the vital link between simulated experiences and real-world clinical practice. Supported by research demonstrating enhanced knowledge, skills, and patient outcomes, effective debriefing mirrors Kolb's experiential learning cycle. Historical roots trace back to World War II, evolving into military after-action reviews and aviation Crew Resource Management training. Modern debriefing emphasizes self-reflection and sustainable performance improvement. Common phases, such as opening the stage, delving deeper, and harvesting learnings, ensure a structured discussion. Techniques like Plus-Delta, Three-Phase Debriefing, and the GAS Model contribute to effective debriefing. Choosing the right debriefing location, be it simulated bedside, a separate room, or in situ simulation, is crucial. The Structured and Supported Debriefing (SSD) model, following the GAS approach, emphasizes structure, support, and participant engagement. Additional tips highlight a humble mindset, ground rules, embracing silence, and lifelong learning. In summary, debriefing is not a post-simulation ritual but the heart of the learning experience, unlocking simulation's potential to empower healthcare professionals, improve patient care, and foster continuous growth.

Keywords Debriefing · GAS model · Supported debriefing · Structured debriefing

Why is debriefing so important? Research shows that simulation, paired with effective debriefing, delivers significant boosts to knowledge, skills, and even patient care outcomes (Levett-Jones & Lapkin, 2014; Niu et al., 2021). It's the bridge between the simulated world and real-world practice, allowing learners to reflect, analyze, and improve their performance.

Consider Kolb's experiential learning cycle (Kolb, 1984): simulation is the concrete experience, and debriefing is the reflection station. Here, participants dissect their actions and thought processes, forming abstract concepts and strategies they can carry into future situations. It's a powerful cycle, and skilled debriefing is the key that unlocks its potential. Skilled debriefers carefully assess the conversation to promote reflection, which allows them to understand the learner's grasp of the concepts and

© The Author(s), under exclusive license to Springer Nature Switzerland AG 2025   67
T. Tangpaisarn et al., *Navigating Healthcare Simulation*,
SpringerBriefs in Education, https://doi.org/10.1007/978-3-031-81265-1_9

can guide the discussion to allow for the continuing discovery of important takeaway points.

9.1 History of Debriefing

During World War II, General Marshall conducted "interviews after combat" with soldiers, not to analyze trauma, but to reconstruct events. This evolved into military "after-action reviews," focused on learning and improving future performance. A series of aviation tragedies fostered the development of Crew Resource Management (CRM) training, where feedback and debriefing became cornerstones. Eventually, full-flight simulators emerged, and by the 1980s, CRM training with skilled facilitators guiding crew debriefings became mandatory across the aviation industry (Gardner, 2013).

Meanwhile, education and psychology offered the concept of facilitation, promoting active learning and aligning with adult learning principles. These diverse roots, including a separate path for trauma-focused Critical Incident Stress Debriefing (CISD), converged to shape our understanding of debriefing in multiple professional fields and, later in healthcare simulation-based education. The emphasis shifted from error-focused critiques to self-reflection, learning, and sustainable performance improvement.

9.2 Common Phases of the Debriefing Process

1. **Opening Stage (Reaction/Description)**:

   (a) **Setting the tone**: Create a safe and supportive environment where participants feel comfortable sharing openly and without judgment. This foundation fosters honest introspection and vulnerability (Abulebda et al., 2023; Gardner, 2013).

   (b) **Establishing goals**: Clearly define the learning objectives of the debriefing session. This clarity ensures everyone is focused on the same target and maximizes the effectiveness of the discussion.

   (c) **Gathering initial impressions**: Invite participants to share their initial thoughts and experiences with the simulation. This provides valuable insights into their individual perspectives and lays the groundwork for deeper analysis.

2. **Delving Deeper (Understanding/Analysis)**:

   (a) **Exploring actions and decisions**: Guide participants into a critical examination of their choices and actions during the simulation. This phase goes beyond surface-level descriptions and encourages self-reflection on why decisions were made and how they impacted the outcome.

(b) **Active questioning**: Facilitate the discussion with probing, open-ended questions that spark deeper thinking and challenge assumptions. Questions like "What were your thought processes?" or "What factors influenced your decision?" ignite introspection and critical analysis.

(c) **Building connections**: Relate the simulated scenario to real-world clinical situations. This bridges the gap between theory and practice, demonstrating the direct applicability of the learning experience.

3. **Harvesting Learnings (Application/Summary)**:

(a) **Summarizing key takeaways**: Distill the most important learnings and insights from the simulation experience and the debriefing. This helps participants solidify their understanding and identify actionable strategies for future practice.

(b) **Formulating strategies**: Encourage participants to translate their newfound knowledge into concrete action plans. This ensures the learning experience doesn't end with the debriefing session but translates into tangible improvements in future clinical performance.

(c) **Planning for the future**: Discuss potential challenges and opportunities for applying the lessons learned in future scenarios. This empowers participants to actively engage in ongoing learning and improvement.

9.3 Common Debriefing Techniques

- **Plus-Delta**: This straightforward approach identifies **strengths (+)** and areas for **improvement (Δ)**. It encourages self-assessment and targeted learning by focusing on both positives and areas for growth.
- **Three-Phase Debriefing**: This structured framework utilizes three phases: **Reaction** (initial impressions), **Analysis** (exploring actions and decisions), and **Summary** (key takeaways and action plans). It provides a clear roadmap for navigating the debriefing journey and ensures all essential elements are covered. Examples of Three-Phase Debriefing include Debriefing with Good Judgment (Rudolph et al., 2006), 3D model (defusing, discovery and deepening) (Zigmont et al., 2011), GAS model (gather, analyze and summarize) (O'Donnell & Phrampus, 2017), and the Diamond debriefing that includes description, analysis, and application (Jaye et al., 2015).
- **Multiphase Debriefing**: Additional phases focused on specific themes (e.g., PEARL, TeamGAINS) (Bajaj et al., 2018; Kolbe et al., 2013).

9.4   GAS Model

The Structured and Supported Debriefing (SSD) model, developed through a collaboration between Winter Institute for Simulation, Education, and Research (WISER) and the American Heart Association (AHA), provides a robust framework for maximizing the educational impact of debriefing across a wide range of healthcare disciplines (O'Donnell & Phrampus, 2017).

Core Principles

- **Structure**: The SSD model follows a three-phase approach: Gather, Analyze, and Summarize (GAS). Each phase has defined goals, facilitator responsibilities, and recommended conversational prompts, ensuring a focused and productive debriefing experience.
- **Support**: SSD recognizes the critical role of both participant well-being and evidence-based learning. It emphasizes emotional debriefing and active participant engagement, facilitating self-reflection and knowledge acquisition. Additionally, the model incorporates external resources such as checklists, algorithms, and best practices as objective sources of truth, reducing tension and fostering learner autonomy.

Phase-Specific Implementation

1. **Gather (G) Phase**:
   (a) **Emotional Safety and Transition**: Prioritize participant well-being by assessing emotional readiness and facilitating decompression from the simulated environment. Encourage active recall of the scenario narrative to establish a shared mental model.
   (b) **Performance Perception Assessment**: Identify any discrepancies between participants' self-perceptions and objective performance (performance gaps) through open-ended questioning and observation. Allows faculty member to help guide participants toward the most important parts of the simulation, as determined by the learning objectives (Table 9.1).

Table 9.1 Performance GAP perception assessment

Facilitator perceptions	Student perceptions		
		Performed well	Performed poorly
	Performed well	Narrow gap Review and reinforce effective behaviors	Wide gap Helping student to understand positive steps in performance
	Performed poorly	Wide gap Helping student to understand problems in performance	Narrow gap Review and correct behaviors that were not effective

2. **Analyze (A) Phase**:

   (a) **Learning Objective Focus**: Guide the discussion towards achieving the predefined learning objectives through targeted questioning and active listening. Encourage participants to analyze their actions, identify areas for improvement, and discover knowledge gaps. Allow learners to cultivate an understanding of how their actions, interactions, performance influenced the outcome of the scenario.

   (b) **Evidence-Based Learning**: Leverage supporting materials such as simulator logs, video recordings, clinical pathways, and institutional guidelines as objective references. This fosters self-discovery, reinforces best practices, and reduces dependence on facilitator expertise.

3. **Summarize (S) Phase**:

   (a) **Key Takeaways and Actionable Insights**: Condense the debriefing into a concise summary, highlighting key learning points and reinforcing their relevance to future clinical practice.

   (b) **Plus-Delta Approach**: Encourage participants to identify two or three "Plus" points (effective actions) and two or three "Delta" points (areas for improvement) through self-reflection. This reinforces positive aspects while promoting targeted improvement strategies.

9.5 Example of Using GAS Model

Gather (G) Phase

- *Facilitator*: "Hi everyone, welcome back from the cardiac arrest scenario. I know it was intense, how are you all feeling?"
- *Learner 1*: "Still a bit shaken, that was close!"
- *Learner 2*: "Yeah, my adrenaline is still pumping."
- *Facilitator*: "Completely understandable. Thanks for sharing that. Can you remind us how the situation unfolded? Who wants to jump in?"
- *Learner 3*: "We found the patient unresponsive, pulseless, not breathing. We immediately started chest compressions and called for backup."
- *Facilitator*: "Excellent recall. What were your initial thoughts and actions?"
- *Learner 1*: "Panic set in for a moment, but I remembered the CABs, so we started CPR, secured the airway, and started rescue breaths."
- *Learner 2*: "I grabbed the defibrillator and attached the pads while we continued compressions."

Analyze (A) Phase

Facilitator: "Fantastic work remembering the CABs under pressure. Let's review the ACLS algorithm. Did we follow the steps correctly in identifying and treating the rhythm?"

Learner 3: "I think so, we recognized ventricular fibrillation and delivered the first shock immediately."

Facilitator: "Right, and what about team communication and role clarity? How did we collaborate effectively under pressure?"

Learner 2: "I could have communicated the defibrillator charge status more clearly before the shock delivery."

Learner 1: "And maybe I could have delegated tasks like managing the bag-valve mask a bit more efficiently."

Facilitator: "Exactly. Now, let's look at the simulator log. Was our compressions depth and rate optimal?"

Learner 3: "Based on the log, maybe we could have focused on deeper compressions during the first few minutes."

Facilitator: "Great observation. Using supporting materials like this is crucial for self-discovery and improvement."

Summarize (S) Phase

Facilitator: "To recap, we learned the importance of: **Quick recognition and action**: Early CPR and prompt defibrillation are critical. **Clear communication and teamwork**: Effective collaboration improves patient outcomes. **Adherence to guidelines**: ACLS algorithms guide efficient and appropriate therapy. **Continuous learning**: Debriefing allows us to reflect and refine our skills."

Facilitator: "Now, let's do the Plus-Delta. What were two things we did effectively (Plus)?"

Learner 1: "Starting CPR immediately and remembering the CABs."

Learner 2: "Prompt defibrillation and coordinating the team effectively."

Facilitator: "And two areas for improvement (Delta)?"

Learner 3: "Deeper compressions initially and clearer communication of AED status."

Learner 2: "Delegating tasks like bag-valve mask management to optimize response."

Facilitator: "Fantastic! This Plus-Delta helps us solidify strengths and identify areas for future practice. Remember, debriefing is a constant learning journey, not a one-time evaluation."

Learner 1: "Thanks for this. It's definitely helpful to analyze what went well and what we can do better next time."

9.6 Adaptability and Impact of GAS Model

The SSD or GAS model's strength lies in its adaptability. Its core principles can be readily applied to various healthcare simulation scenarios, regardless of discipline or complexity (Table 9.2). By adopting SSD, educators can:

- Foster a structured and engaging debriefing environment.
- Promote critical thinking and self-directed learning in participants.

- Create a safe space for reflection on both successes and failures.
- Encourage continuous professional development and improve patient care outcomes.
- Embrace a debriefing model that can be used for any simulation regardless of the complexity.

9.7 Debriefing Locations

Choosing the optimal location for debriefing after a simulation can significantly impact its effectiveness (Phrampus, 2020). Here's a breakdown of three common options, each with its own advantages and considerations:

1. **Simulated Bedside**:

    (a) **Advantages**: Allows participants to remain in the simulated environment, fostering a sense of authenticity and facilitating immediate recall of details. Can emphasize team dynamics and communication within the context of the scenario. Can easily incorporate simulation training equipment into the debriefing discussion.
    (b) **Considerations**: May feel cramped or uncomfortable for larger groups. Potential for disruption if equipment needs resetting. It may not allow participants time or space to decompress from a stressful simulation scenario. Privacy concerns if discussing sensitive topics.

2. **Separate Room**:

    (a) **Advantages**: Provides a dedicated space for focused discussion, free from distractions. Enhances privacy for open dialogue and reflection. Allows easy access to additional resources like guidelines, charts, or videos. The transition to a separate room can give participants time and space to decompress from a stressful simulation scenario. From an operational perspective, it may free up expensive or simulation equipment or environments that are in limited supply.
    (a) **Considerations**: Requires transition from the simulated environment, potentially losing immediacy and momentum. Takes additional time to make the extra transition. May feel disconnected from the scenario context. Might be impractical for in situ simulations.

3. **In Situ Simulation (actual clinical space)**:

    (a) **Advantages**: Offers the highest level of environmental realism, reinforcing context-specific learning within the actual clinical setting. Can be particularly valuable for scenarios involving equipment or workflow unique to that location.

Table 9.2 Summary of GAS model with corresponding goal, actions, sample questions, and time frames

Phase	Goal	Actions	Sample questions	Time frame (%)
Gather	Listen to participants to understand what they think and how they feel about session	Request narrative from team leader	All: Are you feeling ready to begin the debriefing?	25
		Request clarifying or supplemental information from team	Team Leader: Can you tell us what happened when…?	
			Team members: Can you add to the account?	
Analyze	Facilitate participants' reflection on and analysis of their actions	Review of accurate record of events	I noticed…	50
		Report observations (correct and incorrect steps)	Tell me more about…	
		Ask a series of question to reveal participants' thinking processes	How did you feel about…	
		Assist participants to reflect on their performance	What were you thinking when…	
		Direct/redirect participants to assure continuous focus on session objectives	I understand, however, tell me about the "X" aspect of the scenario…	
			Conflict resolution:	
			Let's refocus—"what's important is not who is right but what is right for the patient…"	
Summarize	Facilitate identification and review of lessons learned	Participants identify positive aspects of team or individual behaviors and behaviors that require change	List two actions or events that you felt were effective or well done	25
		Summary of comments or statements	Describe two areas that you think you/ team need to work on…	

(b) **Considerations**: Logistical challenges in clearing space, managing patient traffic, and maintaining sterility. May disrupt ongoing clinical operations. Not always feasible due to space limitations or privacy concerns.

Ultimately, the best debriefing location depends on several factors, including the size, complexity and type of simulation, learning objectives, available resources, and level of disruption to actual clinical environments and personnel (in-situ). Weighing the benefits and drawbacks of each option will help you choose the environment that best promotes an engaging and productive learning experience for your participants. Remember, flexibility is key! Consider combining options, for example, starting with a brief in-situ debriefing to capture immediate emotions and observations, followed by a more detailed discussion in a separate room with access to additional resources.

9.8 Additional Tips for Effective Debriefing

- **Humble mindset**: Approach the debriefing with a humble mindset. Acknowledge your own limitations and be open to learning from participants. This fosters trust and creates a safe space for open dialogue and reflection (Decker et al., 2021; Phrampus, 2021, 2023; Sawyer et al., 2016).
- **Establish Ground Rules**: Set clear expectations for respectful communication, confidentiality, and active participation. This creates a structured environment where everyone feels comfortable contributing.
- **Embrace the Power of Silence**: Give participants time to process questions and formulate their thoughts. Silence is not awkward; it provides valuable space for internal reflection and deeper learning to occur.
- **Balance is Key**: Acknowledge both strengths and areas for improvement. Offer constructive feedback in a supportive manner, highlighting successes while providing actionable steps for future growth.
- **Shared Mental Model**: Ensure everyone agrees on the key events and decisions made during the simulation. This avoids confusion and lays the foundation for constructive analysis.
- **Learning Objectives Revisited**: Reflect on how well the learning objectives were addressed during the debriefing. Use this as an opportunity to identify any gaps or areas needing further exploration.
- **Lifelong Learning Journey**: Acknowledge that learning is a continuous process. Encourage participants to actively seek out opportunities to further develop their skills and knowledge beyond the simulation experience.
- **Non-Judgmental**: While the faculty may judge a p performance to be right or wrong, they should refrain from personalizing the judgement as to why something occurred, or why a particular gap in knowledge may have been discovered.

- **Debriefing Models**: Consider mastering a single debriefing model through repeated practice. As you develop expertise and comfort with debriefing, consider exploring other models that may better suit the learning outcomes you are attempting to achieve.

9.9 Summary

Debriefing is not just a post-simulation formality; it is an important tool within the learning experience provided by simulation. By understanding its core principles, embracing effective techniques, and fostering a nurturing environment, educators can unlock the immense potential of simulation to empower healthcare professionals and ultimately improve patient care. Remember, debriefing is not just a conversation; it is a catalyst for growth, a journey of self-discovery, and, ultimately, the key to unlocking mastery within every simulated experience.

References

Abulebda, K., Auerbach, M., & Limaiem, F. (2023). Debriefing techniques utilized in medical simulation. In: *StatPearls*. StatPearls Publishing. Accessed December 15, 2023. http://www.ncbi.nlm.nih.gov/books/NBK546660/

Bajaj, K., Meguerdichian, M., Thoma, B., Huang, S., Eppich, W., & Cheng, A. (2018). The PEARLS healthcare debriefing tool. *Academic Medicine, 93*(2), 336. https://doi.org/10.1097/ACM.0000000000002035

Decker, S., Alinier, G., Crawford, S. B., Gordon, R. M., Jenkins, D., & Wilson, C. (2021). Healthcare simulation standards of best Practice™ the debriefing process. *Clinical Simulation in Nursing, 58*, 27–32. https://doi.org/10.1016/j.ecns.2021.08.011

Gardner, R. (2013). Introduction to debriefing. *Seminars in Perinatology, 37*(3), 166–174. https://doi.org/10.1053/j.semperi.2013.02.008

Jaye, P., Thomas, L., & Reedy, G. (2015). "The Diamond": A structure for simulation debrief. *The Clinical Teacher, 12*(3), 171–175. https://doi.org/10.1111/tct.12300

Kolb, D. (1984). *Experiential learning: Experience as the source of learning and development* (Vol. 1).

Kolbe, M., Weiss, M., Grote, G., et al. (2013). TeamGAINS: A tool for structured debriefings for simulation-based team trainings. *BMJ Quality and Safety, 22*(7), 541–553. https://doi.org/10.1136/bmjqs-2012-000917

Levett-Jones, T., & Lapkin, S. (2014). A systematic review of the effectiveness of simulation debriefing in health professional education. *Nurse Education Today, 34*(6), e58-63. https://doi.org/10.1016/j.nedt.2013.09.020

Niu, Y., Liu, T., Li, K., et al. (2021). Effectiveness of simulation debriefing methods in nursing education: A systematic review and meta-analysis. *Nurse Education Today, 107*, 105113. https://doi.org/10.1016/j.nedt.2021.105113

O'Donnell, J., & Phrampus, P. (2017). Simulation in nurse anesthesia. In B. Henrich & J. Thompson (Eds.), *A resource for nurse anesthesia educators* (2nd ed., pp. 261–294). American Association of Nurse Anesthetists.

Phrampus, P. E. (2020, May 22). Where do we debrief? *Simulating Healthcare*. A blog dedicated to discussions and relevant things regarding simulation in healthcare in healthcare. Accessed January 2, 2024. https://simulatinghealthcare.net/2020/05/22/where-do-we-debrief/

Phrampus, P. E. (2021, September 21). Five tips for creating hybrid curricula for simulation based learning. *Simulating Healthcare*. A blog dedicated to discussions and relevant things regarding simulation in healthcare in healthcare. Accessed December 4, 2023. https://simulatinghealthcare.net/2021/09/21/five-tips-for-creating-hybrid-curricula-for-simulation-based-learning/

Phrampus, P. E. (2023, August 8). HUMBLE—Six traits for better simulation and debriefing. *Simulating Healthcare*. Accessed January 2, 2024. https://simulatinghealthcare.net/2023/08/08/humble-six-traits-that-will-make-you-a-better-simulation-educator-and-lead-effective-debriefings/

Rudolph, J. W., Simon, R., Dufresne, R. L., & Raemer, D. B. (2006). There's no such thing as "non-judgmental" debriefing: A theory and method for debriefing with good judgment. *Simulation in Healthcare, 1*(1), 49–55. https://doi.org/10.1097/01266021-200600110-00006

Sawyer, T., Eppich, W., Brett-Fleegler, M., Grant, V., & Cheng, A. (2016). More than one way to debrief: A critical review of healthcare simulation debriefing methods. *Simulation in Healthcare, 11*(3), 209. https://doi.org/10.1097/SIH.0000000000000148

Zigmont, J. J., Kappus, L. J., & Sudikoff, S. N. (2011). The 3D model of debriefing: Defusing, discovering, and deepening. *Seminars in Perinatology, 35*(2), 52–58. https://doi.org/10.1053/j.semperi.2011.01.003

Chapter 10
Learner Assessment

Abstract The chapter highlights formative, summative, and high-stakes assessments in simulation, emphasizing their roles in enhancing clinical competence. Assessment tools like checklists, rating scales, and rubrics are detailed, with characteristics for each. The importance of validity and reliability in simulation assessment is discussed, with insights into construct, content, and criterion validity, along with test-retest, interrater, and internal consistency reliability. Practical tips for ensuring validity and reliability are provided. The chapter concludes by underscoring the pivotal role of effective assessment in maximizing educational benefits in healthcare simulation.

Keywords Formative assessment · Summative assessment · High-stakes assessment · Assessment tools

For this chapter, assessment refers to an analysis of learners' performance during a simulation that helps to determine whether or not the simulation scenario was successfully completed. Assessment can take various forms, ranging from the opinion of the faculty member to the development of simple assessment tools or, at times, more complex assessment tools and methods that may be required depending on the overall objectives of the simulation activity.

10.1 Purposes of Assessment

The purposes of assessment during simulations may range from being able to improve performance through coaching (formative), or perhaps delivering a grade that quantifies the performance (summative). Additionally, and possibly unrelated to specific learner outcomes in the scenario, assessments within a simulation may be incorporated as a component of research projects. For example, there may be interest in researching the impact of design element changes on the efficiency or effectiveness of a simulation activity (Kardong-Edgren et al., 2022; McMahon et al., 2021).

T. Tangpaisarn et al., *Navigating Healthcare Simulation*,
SpringerBriefs in Education, https://doi.org/10.1007/978-3-031-81265-1_10

1. **Formative Assessment**

Formative assessment in healthcare simulation involves feedback during the learning process. It provides learners with insights into their performance, allowing for immediate adjustments and improvements. In simulated scenarios, formative assessment can take the form of real-time feedback from instructors, encouraging reflection and skill refinement.

2. **Summative Assessment**

Summative assessment is generally completed at the conclusion of a simulation session or course, but data may be gathered throughout the simulation. It aims to evaluate the overall performance and competence of learners. Summative assessments may include scenario-based evaluations, objective structured clinical examinations (OSCEs), or other structured evaluations to gauge the achievement of specific learning outcomes.

3. **High-Stakes Assessment**

High-stakes assessments are critical evaluations that **have significant consequences** for learners. In healthcare simulation, these assessments may mimic real-world scenarios and are often used to assess readiness for clinical practice. High-stakes assessments contribute to ensuring that healthcare professionals are well-prepared to handle complex situations in a clinical setting.

10.2   Common Types of Assessment Tools

10.2.1   Checklists

Checklists, acting as a systematic process measure, ensure all essential steps or actions are completed. They reflect best practices and are ideal for beginners or tasks with clear, defined steps. Their strength lies in enhanced consistency in evaluation (reliability). However, their binary nature (completed/not completed) can limit their ability to capture the full picture of whether the performance truly represents what was intended to be measured (validity) (McLaughlin, 2010; Vesterinen, 2023) (Table 10.1).

10.2.2   Characteristics of Good Checklists

- **Structured**: Checklists consist of a set of predefined criteria or steps that participants are expected to perform during the simulation. These criteria are usually specific, observable, and measurable actions.

Table 10.1 Example of using a checklist as an assessment tool during ultrasound guided central venous catheter insertion simulation (*courtesy* WISER)

Name	
	☑
1. **Consent the patient,** identify allergies (lidocaine, latex, heparin)	
2. **Wash hands**	
3. **Assemble and verify proper procedure kit, ultrasound, ultrasound sterile probe cover**	
4. **Prior to cleaning, identify location with ultrasound,** assessing for IJ collapsibility and patency, location near carotid artery—below the bifurcation, where the vein does not overlap the artery	
5. **Mark location with skin marker**	
6. **Proper positioning of patient** **Orientation of bed and supplies tray** **Organization of equipment (need all 3/3)**	
7. **Open tray without contamination**	
8. **Don maximum sterile barriers (must have all elements)**	
(a) Ensure all assistants have hat and masks	
(b) Put on Hat, mask, sterile gown, sterile gloves, eye protection	
(c) Organize open sterile tray	
(d) Skin prep x3 with Betadine, or other approved solution, allow site to dry for 30 s	
(e) Position sterile drape over entire patient's body, properly positioned	
(f) Once sterile, with assistance place ultrasound probe within sterile cover. Secure probe	
(g) Review syringe and needle, guidewire mobility within introducer	

- **Task-Oriented**: They are particularly effective for assessing procedural skills and adherence to protocols. Each item on the checklist corresponds to a task or action that is critical to the successful completion of the simulation scenario.
- **Objective and Quantifiable**: Checklists facilitate objective and quantifiable assessments. Assessors can mark off each criterion as it is completed, providing a clear record of the participant's performance.
- **Quick and Efficient**: Checklists are designed for efficiency. They allow assessors to quickly and systematically evaluate participants, making them suitable for scenarios with time constraints or when assessing multiple participants.
- **Standardization**: Checklists contribute to standardizing the assessment process. By clearly defining the criteria for success, they help ensure consistency in evaluations across different assessors and simulation sessions.
- **Usability Improvements**: Basic usability improvements, such as readable fonts, avoiding ALL CAPS, and enhancing contrast, contribute to better user perception and expectancy of the task steps.

Table 10.2 Example of using a rating scale as the assessment tool

	Unacceptable		Average		Above expectations
Communications skills	1	2	3	4	5
History taking	1	2	3	4	5
Physical examination	1	2	3	4	5
Treatment	1	2	3	4	5

10.2.3   Rating Scales

Rating scales judge the outcome of a performance. They should be based on agreed-upon criteria (consensus) and are most effective for advanced learners tackling complex tasks. Rating scales excel at assessing quality and differentiating performance levels, offering greater validity. However, their reliance on subjective judgment can lead to lower reliability compared to checklists (https://tgm.academy/tips-for-effectively-designing-rating-scale.html) (Table 10.2).

10.2.4   Characteristics of Good Rating Scales

- **Graduated Scale**: Rating scales consist of a graduated scale, typically ranging from low to high or poor to excellent. Each point on the scale represents a different level of performance or proficiency.
- **Behavioral Descriptors**: Each point on the scale is associated with behavioral descriptors that guide assessors in assigning scores. These descriptors help standardize the assessment process and ensure consistency among different assessors.
- **Balanced Scale**: Maintain a balanced distribution of levels to avoid a skewed assessment. If possible, use an odd number of levels to include a midpoint.
- **Focus on Observable Behaviors**: Frame criteria in terms of observable behaviors rather than inferred traits. This enhances objectivity and ensures assessors can make clear observations.
- **Align with Learning Objectives**: Ensure that the rating scale aligns with the learning objectives of the assessment. This connection enhances the validity of the assessment.
- **Encourage Feedback**: Often times rating scales are used to provide a mechanism for assessors to provide constructive feedback to the individuals being assessed. This promotes a growth-oriented approach to assessment.

10.2.5   Rubric Scales

Rubrics provide a structured framework for evaluating performance across multiple criteria. They typically consist of a grid with specific criteria listed on one axis and performance levels (e.g., excellent, proficient, needs improvement) on the other. Each cell within the grid describes what successful performance looks like at each level. This detailed breakdown offers a clear picture of strengths and weaknesses, making rubrics valuable for both formative assessment (providing ongoing feedback) and summative assessment (assigning a final grade). While rubrics require more time to develop, they can be highly effective for tasks with defined criteria and desired learning outcomes (https://teaching-resources.delta.ncsu. edu/rubric_best-practices-examples-templates/; https://www.niu.edu/citl/resources/ guides/instructional-guide/rubrics-for-assessment.shtml; Jonsson & Svingby, 2007; Reddy & Andrade, 2010) (Table 10.3).

Table 10.3 Example of a Rubric-based assessment tool

Criteria	Excellent (4 pts)	Good (3 pts)	Fair (2 pts)	Poor (1 pt)
Scene safety	Checks scene for safety hazards and secures the scene	Checks scene but may miss minor hazards	Does not fully check scene for safety	Does not check scene for safety
Rescuer assessment	Checks responsiveness using "Shake and Shout" technique	Checks responsiveness but technique may be weak	May not check responsiveness or technique is incorrect	Does not check responsiveness
Breathing and pulse check	Checks for breathing (look, listen, feel) and pulse for a limited time (no more than 10 s)	Checks for breathing and pulse but technique may be slow or incomplete	May not check for breathing or pulse or technique is incorrect	Does not check for breathing or pulse
Compression depth and rate	Performs compressions at least 2 inches (5 cm) deep at a rate of 100–120 per minute	Performs compressions with somewhat adequate depth (1.5–2 inches) and rate (90–100 per minute)	Performs compressions with inadequate depth or rate	Does not perform compressions or compressions are ineffective
Hand placement	Hands are placed correctly on the lower half of the sternum	Hand placement may be slightly off-center	Hand placement is significantly off-center	Hands are not placed on the sternum

10.2.6   Characteristics of Good Rubric Scales

- **Clearly Define Criteria**: Clearly articulate the criteria or dimensions that you want to assess. These criteria should align with the learning objectives or outcomes you intend to measure.
- **Identify Levels of Proficiency**: Define distinct levels of proficiency for each criterion. Commonly, a 3–5-point scale is used, but the number of levels may vary based on the complexity of the assessment.
- **Use Descriptive Language**: Use descriptive language for each level of proficiency. Clearly communicate what distinguishes one level from another. Avoid vague or subjective terms.
- **Provide Clear Examples**: Include clear examples or descriptors for each level of proficiency. These examples should illustrate the expected performance at each level and guide assessors in their evaluations.
- **Focus on Measurable Outcomes**: Ensure that each criterion and level of proficiency corresponds to measurable outcomes. This enhances objectivity and makes assessments more reliable.
- **Balance Positive and Negative Descriptors**: Maintain a balanced approach in your language. Include both positive and negative descriptors to ensure fairness and completeness in the evaluation.
- **Align with Learning Objectives**: Ensure that the rubric aligns with the learning objectives or outcomes of the assessment. This alignment enhances the validity of the rubric.

10.3   Ensuring Validity and Reliability

10.3.1   Validity

Validity refers to the degree to which an assessment tool or instrument measures what it is intended to measure. In the context of healthcare simulation, validity ensures that the assessment accurately evaluates the targeted skills, behaviors, or competencies (American Educational Research Association, American Psychological Association & National Council on Measurement in Education, 2014; Chiang et al., 2015; Jonsson & Svingby, 2007; Middleton, 2019; Moskal, 2000).

The validity of assessments can be evaluated through three key types of evidence.

1. **Construct Validity**: The degree to which an **assessment aligns with existing theories and knowledge** related to the simulated scenario or skills being measured.
2. **Content Validity**: Ensuring the assessment **covers all essential aspects** of the concepts being measured.
3. **Criterion Validity**: Make sure the assessment **correspond to other** valid measures of the same healthcare concepts.

10.3.2 Ensuring Validity in Healthcare Simulation

- Clearly define the learning objectives and outcomes.
- Involve subject matter experts in the development and review of simulation scenarios and assessment tools.
- Use a variety of assessment methods to triangulate information and enhance the validity of the overall assessment process.

10.3.3 Reliability

Reliability refers to the consistency, stability, and dependability of assessment results. A reliable assessment tool should produce consistent outcomes when applied to the same scenario, skill, or performance over time. The following types of reliability assessments provide dependability and accuracy of healthcare simulation assessments (American Educational Research Association, American Psychological Association & National Council on Measurement in Education, 2014; Chiang et al., 2015; Jonsson & Svingby, 2007; Middleton, 2019; Moskal, 2000):

1. **Test–Retest Reliability**: Examines the consistency of a measurement **across time**. It addresses whether the same results are obtained when the simulation scenario or assessment is repeated.
2. **Interrater Reliability**: Assesses the consistency of measurement **across different assessors or observers**. It explores whether the same results are obtained when different individuals conduct the same simulation assessment.
3. **Internal Consistency Reliability**: Evaluates the **consistency of the measurement itself** within a simulation scenario. It investigates whether the same results are obtained from different aspects of the simulation designed to measure the same healthcare competencies.

10.3.4 Ensuring Reliability in Healthcare Simulation

- Provide standardized training for assessors to ensure a common understanding of assessment criteria (Phrampus, 2022).
- Clearly define scoring criteria and guidelines to minimize subjectivity.
- Regularly monitor and assess inter-rater reliability through calibration sessions and discussions among assessors.
- Consider Video Scoring to significantly improve scoring accuracy and interrater reliability.

10.4 Summary

In conclusion, effective assessment in healthcare simulation is crucial for shaping competent and confident learners. Incorporating formative and summative assessments, utilizing various assessment tools, and ensuring the validity and reliability of evaluations contribute to the success of simulation-based learning experiences. As healthcare simulation continues to evolve, thoughtful assessment practices play a pivotal role in maximizing the educational benefits for learners.

References

American Educational Research Association, American Psychological Association, National Council on Measurement in Education (Eds.). (2014). *Standards for educational and psychological testing.* American Educational Research Association.

Chiang, I. C. A., Jhangiani, R. S., & Price, P. C. (2015, October 13). *Reliability and validity of measurement.* Accessed January 10, 2024. https://opentextbc.ca/researchmethods/chapter/reliability-and-validity-of-measurement/

Jonsson, A., & Svingby, G. (2007). The use of scoring rubrics: Reliability, validity and educational consequences. *Educational Research Review, 2*(2), 130–144. https://doi.org/10.1016/j.edurev.2007.05.002

Kardong-Edgren, S., Swiderski, D., Noland, H., Wasseem, M., Charles, S., & Chen, S. (2022). *CHSE blueprint review reference manual.* Society for Simulation in Healthcare.

McLaughlin, A. C. (2010, October 1). *What makes a good checklist.* Accessed January 13, 2024. https://psnet.ahrq.gov/perspective/what-makes-good-checklist

McMahon, E., Jimenez, F. A., Lawrence, K., & Victor, J. (2021). Healthcare Simulation Standards of Best Practice™ evaluation of learning and performance. *Clinical Simulation in Nursing, 58*, 54–56. https://doi.org/10.1016/j.ecns.2021.08.016

Middleton, F. (2019, July 3). Reliability vs. validity in research I Difference, types and examples. *Scribbr.* Accessed January 10, 2024. https://www.scribbr.com/methodology/reliability-vs-validity/

Moskal, B., & Leydens, J. (2000). Scoring Rubric development: Validity and reliability. *Practical Assessment Research and Evaluation, 7.*

Phrampus, P. E. (2022, June 6). 5 tips to improve interrater reliability during healthcare simulation assessments. *Simulating Healthcare. A blog dedicated to discussions and relevant things regarding simulation in healthcare in healthcare.* Accessed January 5, 2024. https://simulatinghealthcare.net/2022/06/06/5-tips-to-improve-interrater-reliability-during-healthcare-simulation-assessments/

Reddy, Y. M., & Andrade, H. (2010). A review of rubric use in higher education. *Assessment & Evaluation in Higher Education, 35*(4), 435–448. https://doi.org/10.1080/02602930902862859

Rubric best practices, examples, and templates—Teaching resources. Accessed January 13, 2024. https://teaching-resources.delta.ncsu.edu/rubric_best-practices-examples-templates/

Rubrics for Assessment I Center for Innovative Teaching and Learning. Northern Illinois University. Accessed January 13, 2024. https://www.niu.edu/citl/resources/guides/instructional-guide/rubrics-for-assessment.shtml

Tips for designing a rating scale I TGM Academy. Accessed January 13, 2024. https://tgm.academy/tips-for-effectively-designing-rating-scale.html

Vesterinen, K. (2023, February 7). *5 tips for creating great checklists.* Accessed January 12, 2024. https://blog.falcony.io/en/tips-for-great-checklists

Chapter 11
Healthcare Simulation Program Evaluation

Abstract This chapter emphasizes the critical role of continuous quality improvement in healthcare simulation programs through effective evaluation. Program evaluation at various levels—program, course, or scenario—helps identify areas of need and ensures the program aligns with stakeholders' needs. Key constituents for feedback include learners, faculty, staff, and the organization, each offering unique insights that drive program enhancement. Learner feedback improves simulation effectiveness, empowers students, and supports evidence-based innovation. Faculty perspectives ensure the accuracy and clinical relevance of simulations, while staff feedback addresses logistical improvements for a seamless learning experience. Evaluating program facilities ensures an optimal learning environment, while organizational perception aligns the simulation program with institutional goals and supports accreditation. Additionally, tools developed by Kim Leighton and her team offer valuable psychometrically tested instruments for evaluating various facets of simulation-based education. By integrating these feedback mechanisms, healthcare simulation programs can continually improve their educational value, operational efficiency, and contribution to better healthcare outcomes.

Keywords Healthcare simulation · Program evaluation · Continuous quality improvement · Stakeholder feedback · Simulation effectiveness

Establishing a healthy culture of continuous quality improvement is beneficial for healthcare simulation programs. A tool of continuous quality improvement that should be considered is the evaluation of the simulation program itself. This can be done at the program level, the course level, or even at the scenario level. Carefully identifying the stakeholders, resources, and people involved in carrying out a successful mission can help guide the structure of a quality improvement program. The importance of this is highlighted in the Society for Simulation Healthcare's accreditation program requirements (https://www.ssih.org/Portals/48/2021%20SSH%20TEACHING-EDUCAT ION%20STANDARDS%20COMPANION%20DOCUMENT_1.pdf).

T. Tangpaisarn et al., *Navigating Healthcare Simulation*,
SpringerBriefs in Education, https://doi.org/10.1007/978-3-031-81265-1_11

Program evaluation can be targeted at areas of suspected need for improvement or established broadly for ongoing surveillance of aspects of quality of the program. Common constituents that are the focus of the evaluation include learners of the simulation programs, the faculty who carry out the programs, as well as the staff of the simulation center. Additionally, evaluation of the program could include broader constituents of the parent organization to assess the perception that the simulation program is capable of contributing to the needs of the organization. Receiving feedback from various stakeholders is essential for the following reasons:

Student Feedback

- **Improves Simulation Effectiveness**:
    - Provides direct insights into how well simulations meet learning objectives.
    - Identifies strengths and weaknesses in scenarios, instructional techniques, and curriculum integration.

- **Empowers Learners**:
    - Values student opinions and experiences.
    - Tailors simulations to real-world clinical challenges.
    - Increases educational value and relevance.

- **Drives Quality Improvement**:
    - Fosters a culture of continuous improvement and innovation.
    - Encourages evidence-based practices and innovative teaching methods.

- **Identifies Areas for Enhancement**:
    - Reveals trends and patterns in student feedback.
    - Guides modifications to simulation design, scenario content, and technological infrastructure.

- **Ensures Best Practices**:
    - Helps programs comply with best educational practices.
    - Maintains program dynamism and responsiveness to evolving needs.

Faculty Feedback

- **Expertise in Curriculum and Clinical Practice**:
    - Assess how simulations integrate with the broader curriculum.
    - Evaluate the accuracy of simulations in replicating real-life scenarios.

- **Dual Perspective**:
    - Balance educational theory with practical application.

- **Maintains Program Rigor and Relevance**:
    - Ensures simulations are methodologically sound and clinically relevant.
    - Makes simulations more effective teaching tools reflecting actual challenges.

- **Drives Continuous Improvement**:
  - Guides advancements in teaching methods, simulation technologies, and scenario development.
  - Identifies areas where simulations can be improved to prepare students for real-world settings.

- **Innovation and Adaptability**:
  - Suggests improvements and creates new scenarios for emerging medical issues and advancements.
  - Helps programs keep pace with the evolving healthcare landscape.

- **Prepares Students for Future Roles**:
  - Ensures simulations remain relevant and prepare students effectively for their careers.

Staff Feedback

- **Unique Perspective on Logistics and Operations**:
  - Offer insights into equipment usability, resource adequacy, and simulation environment effectiveness.

- **Ensures Seamless Learning Experience**:
  - Identifies logistical and technical inefficiencies that disrupt student learning.

- **Highlights Overlooked Improvement Areas**:
  - Points out practical challenges in setup, breakdown, and workflow.

- **Informs Quality Improvement Strategies**:
  - Recommends upgrades for simulation technologies and facilities.
  - Improves operational efficiency and reduces downtime.

- **Creates an Optimal Learning Environment**:
  - Integrates feedback on both educational tools and participant dynamics.
  - Fosters a realistic and conducive learning environment reflecting clinical settings.

Feedback on Simulation Program Facilities

- **Ensures Effective Learning Environment**:
  - Evaluates if facilities (physical spaces & technology) meet educational needs and learning outcomes.
  - Identifies issues with space limitations, equipment, or aesthetics impacting engagement and comfort.

- **Improves Learner Experience**:
    - Gauges how well facilities support or hinder the simulation experience.

- **Drives Quality Improvement**:
    - Ensures infrastructure keeps pace with evolving education and technology.
    - Maintains adherence to safety and accessibility standards.

- **Informs Strategic Investments**:
    - Feedback guides the process for upgrades in simulation equipment and layout design.

- **Enhances Overall Program Quality**:
    - Leads to more effective and efficient training sessions.
    - Improves the quality of healthcare education provided.

- **Supports Continuous Improvement**:
    - Feedback integration informs quality improvement plans.
    - Better serve the educational needs of healthcare professionals and organizations.

Organizational Perception

- **Aligns Program with Institutional Goals**:
    - Gathers feedback on how the institution views the program's effectiveness in education, operations, and contribution to clinical training, research, and patient care.
    - Helps understand if the program is considered a valuable asset meeting departmental needs.

- **Justifies Continued Support**:
    - Informs decisions on funding, personnel, space allocation, and curriculum integration.
    - Showcases program achievements and impact to secure its role within the institution.

- **Guides Strategic Planning**:
    - Identifies areas for improvement or expansion, like introducing new technologies or scenarios.

- **Supports Accreditation Processes**:
    - Demonstrates institutional engagement and adherence to educational standards.

- **Enhances Program Reputation and Effectiveness**:
  - Aligns program with the institution's mission and healthcare education advancements.
  - Strengthens the program's position within the institution.
- **Contributes to Improved Healthcare Outcomes**:
  - Feedback loop ensures program efforts contribute to better quality and safety in healthcare

Extending beyond the typical learner assessment and program evaluation, Kim Leighton and her research team have developed a series of useful evaluation instruments for healthcare simulation educators and researchers. These instruments have been designed to evaluate various aspects of simulation-based education. These instruments include the simulation culture organizational readiness, simulation educator needs assessment, clinical learning environment comparison survey, facilitator competency, and simulation effectiveness. It is worth noting that all of these instruments have undergone psychometric testing, ensuring their validity and reliability as evaluation methods for healthcare simulation. Even better, these instruments are freely available for anyone to access. You can find them at (https://www.health ysimulation.com/tools/evaluating-healthcare-simulation/).

References

Evaluating Healthcare Simulation I Healthcare Simulation I HealthySimulation.com. Published October 1, 2023. Accessed February 4, 2024. https://www.healthysimulation.com/tools/evaluating-healthcare-simulation/

Society for Simulation in Healthcare. Committee for Accreditation of Healthcare Simulation Programs Teaching/Education Accreditation Standards Companion Document. https://www.ssih.org/Portals/48/2021%20SSH%20TEACHING-EDUCATION%20STANDARDS%20COMPANION%20DOCUMENT_1.pdf

Chapter 12
Interprofessional Education (IPE)

Abstract Interprofessional Education (IPE) serves as a foundational step toward fostering interprofessional collaborative practice among healthcare professionals. It involves learners from multiple professions engaging in shared learning experiences, promoting effective collaboration and ultimately improving patient outcomes. The Interprofessional Education Collaborative (IPEC) has outlined four core competencies for interprofessional collaborative practice, emphasizing values, ethics, roles, responsibilities, communication, and teamwork. The unique characteristics of IPE simulations, as distinguished from single-profession simulations, lie in their objectives, content, and learner interactions, with a focus on interdisciplinary teamwork, communication, and shared decision-making. In addition to considering key differences, successful IPE simulations involve interdisciplinary collaboration in scenario development, pre-briefing on collaboration, and dedicated debriefing sessions. The benefits of IPE simulations include improved patient safety, enhanced interdisciplinary understanding, realistic skill application, and professional networking. Despite its advantages, IPE simulation faces challenges such as scheduling conflicts and logistical issues, requiring institutional commitment and innovative solutions for long-term success. Overall, IPE simulation plays a pivotal role in shaping a collaborative healthcare workforce that prioritizes patient-centered care and effective teamwork.

Keywords Interprofessional · Collaboration · Patient outcomes · Teamwork · Communication

Interprofessional Education (IPE) of healthcare professionals is aimed to be an important part of establishing interprofessional collaborative practice (IPCP). IPE occurs when learners from two or more professions learn about, from, and with each other to enable effective collaboration and improve health outcomes. Once learners understand how to work interprofessional, they are ready to enter the workplace as members of the collaborative practice team. Simulation can play an important role in IPE. This is a crucial step in moving health systems from fragmentation to a position of strength (World Health Organization (WHO) 2010).

12.1   Core Competencies of IPE Simulation

In the United States, six national education associations representing schools of the health professions (allopathic medicine, osteopathic medicine, dentistry, nursing, pharmacy, and public health) have formed a collaborative called the Interprofessional Education Collaborative (IPEC). Their mission is to promote and encourage efforts by member organizations to advance meaningful interprofessional learning experiences. These experiences aim to prepare future health professionals for enhanced team-based care of patients and improved population health outcomes. IPEC first published the core competencies for interprofessional collaborative practice in 2011, which were recently updated in 2023 (Interprofessional Education Collaborative, 2023). Below are the four core competencies for interprofessional collaborative practice.

1. **Values and Ethics**: Work with team members to maintain a climate of shared values, ethical conduct, and mutual respect.
2. **Roles and Responsibilities**: Use the knowledge of one's role and team members' expertise to address individual and population health outcomes.
3. **Communication**: Communicate in a responsive, responsible, respectful, and compassionate manner with team members.
4. **Teams and Teamwork**: Apply values and principles of the science of teamwork to adapt one's role in various team settings.

These competencies are an integral part of interprofessional collaboration and ensure that patient and family-centered care is provided while keeping in mind the needs of the community and population.

12.2   Key Difference in IPE Simulation

While scenario design principles apply to both single profession and IPE simulations, the focus and objectives shift significantly when fostering interdisciplinary collaboration (Boet et al., 2014; Rossler et al., 2021). Team Strategies and Tools to Enhance Performance and Patient Safety (TeamSTEPPS®) is an example of a curriculum that provides an evidence-based framework to optimize team performance across the healthcare delivery system (https://www.ahrq.gov/teamstepps-program/index.html). Table 12.1 shows the key differences between a single profession and IPE simulation.

It should be noted that higher success will be achieved by designing the simulation scenario for interprofessional education as a sole focus from the onset, as opposed to repurposing an old scenario design for individual simulation.

Table 12.1 Key difference between single profession and IPE simulation

Feature	Single profession simulation	IPE simulation
Objectives	Develop individual skills, decision-making, and procedural proficiency within a discipline	Foster interdisciplinary teamwork, communication, and shared decision-making for patient-centered care
Content and context	Covers a wide range of clinical scenarios within a specific discipline	Requires input and collaboration from multiple disciplines, reflecting real-world team situations
Learner roles and interactions	Primarily interactions with standardized patients or mannequins, focusing on individual performance	Active interactions between learners playing designated professional roles, promoting communication and collaboration

12.3 Additional Consideration for IPE Simulation

- **Involve interdisciplinary team members**: Engage healthcare professionals from different disciplines in scenario development and facilitation to ensure authenticity and diverse perspectives (Boet et al., 2014; https://www.ahrq.gov/teamstepps-program/index.html).
- **Pre-brief learners on collaboration**: Prepare learners for their roles and emphasize the importance of interprofessional communication and teamwork, which may utilize the TeamSTEPPS® approach.
- **Debriefing**: Dedicate time for debriefing, focusing not just on clinical skills but also on team dynamics, communication effectiveness, and conflict resolution strategies, which can also utilize the TeamSTEPPS® approach.

12.4 Benefits of IPE Simulation

- **Improved patient safety**: By enhancing teamwork and communication skills in a simulated environment, IPE contributes to enhanced patient safety. Healthcare professionals work collaboratively are better equipped to prevent errors, respond to emergencies, and provide optimal care (Pinar, 2015).
- **Enhanced interdisciplinary understanding**: IPE simulations break down stereotypes and misconceptions about other healthcare professions. Through shared experiences, participants gain a deeper understanding of the roles and responsibilities of their interprofessional colleagues, fostering a culture of mutual respect.

- **Realistic skill application**: IPE simulations allow participants to apply their skills and knowledge in scenarios that closely resemble real-world situations. This realistic application enhances their ability to adapt to dynamic healthcare environments and collaborate seamlessly.
- **Professional networking**: IPE simulations allow learners to build professional connections early in their education. Establishing relationships with peers from different disciplines can lead to a network of collaborative healthcare professionals, creating a supportive community for future practice.

12.5 Challenges

While IPE simulation brings numerous benefits, challenges such as scheduling conflicts, logistical issues, and the need for dedicated resources may arise. Addressing these challenges requires institutional commitment, innovative solutions, and recognition of the long-term benefits for both learners and the healthcare system (Boet et al., 2014).

Novice debriefers can be challenged by staying focused on IPE, as there is a tendency for them to regress towards covering topics associated with clinical skill competency.

12.6 Summary

IPE simulation is a cornerstone in shaping the next generation of collaborative healthcare professionals. By integrating diverse perspectives, fostering effective communication, and emphasizing patient-centered care, IPE simulations pave the way for a healthcare workforce that thrives on collaboration, ultimately benefiting patients worldwide.

References

Boet, S., Bould, M. D., Layat Burn, C., & Reeves, S. (2014). Twelve tips for a successful interprofessional team-based high-technology simulation education session. *Medical Teacher, 36*(10), 853–857. https://doi.org/10.3109/0142159X.2014.923558

Interprofessional Education Collaborative. (2023). *IPEC core competencies for interprofessional collaborative practice: version 3*. Interprofessional Education Collaborative.

Pinar, G. (2015). Simulation-enhanced interprofessional education in health care. *Creative Education, 6*(17), 1852–1859. https://doi.org/10.4236/ce.2015.617189

Rossler, K., Molloy, M. A., Pastva, A. M., Brown, M., & Xavier, N. (2021). Healthcare Simulation Standards of Best Practice™ simulation-enhanced interprofessional education. *Clinical Simulation in Nursing, 58*, 49–53. https://doi.org/10.1016/j.ecns.2021.08.015

TeamSTEPPS Pocket Guide and App. Accessed February 16, 2024. https://www.ahrq.gov/teamst epps-program/resources/pocket-guide/index.html

TeamSTEPPS (Team Strategies & Tools to Enhance Performance & Patient Safety). Accessed February 7, 2024. https://www.ahrq.gov/teamstepps-program/index.html

World Health Organization (WHO). (2010). *Framework for action on interprofessional education & collaborative practice*. World Health Organization.

Chapter 13
Strategies to Engage Professional Colleagues in Healthcare Simulation

Abstract This chapter explores strategies for effectively engaging professional colleagues in healthcare simulation, a crucial aspect of promoting meaningful learning experiences. Recognizing the importance of collaboration among healthcare professionals in simulation initiatives, the chapter delves into innovative approaches to gather active participation. The narrative emphasizes the significance of aligning simulation activities with the specific needs and interests of diverse healthcare disciplines. Key strategies discussed include fostering a culture of inclusivity, tailoring simulations to address profession-specific challenges, and utilizing technology to enhance engagement. The chapter also highlights the role of effective communication and collaboration in building a supportive community of practice. By offering insights into successful methods and addressing potential challenges, this chapter aims to provide a valuable resource for educators, simulation facilitators, and healthcare professionals seeking to optimize engagement in simulation-based learning.

Keywords Engaging · Inclusivity · Profession-specific challenges · Colleagues

Healthcare simulation offers a powerful tool for enhancing clinical skills, fostering teamwork, and improving patient outcomes. However, successfully integrating simulation into the organization requires acquiring the necessary resources and garnering your colleagues' active participation to serve in the role of faculty. Key strategies that WISER uses to overcome the challenges and empower healthcare professionals to embrace simulation-based learning are expressed below (https://www.wisersimulation.org/news/).

Demonstrating the Value to Leadership

- **Speak the executive leader's language**: Translate simulation's benefits into terms that resonate with leadership. Highlight potential cost savings through improved efficiency, reduced errors, and enhanced patient safety. Showcase how simulation aligns with strategic goals for improved quality of care and professional development. Ensure there is alignment between the simulation program and the sponsoring organization's quality and safety goals.

- **Gather data and share success stories**: If you already have a simulation program, present concrete data on its positive impact. Quantify improvements in areas that align with the organizations goals such as focused patient safety initiates like difficult airway management, central venous access issues and catheter associated urinary tract infections. Look for other opportunities that align with active quality improvement programs that the institution may be working on such as team communication in the operating room or patient satisfaction. Share compelling testimonials from participants who have benefited from the experience. At WISER, a periodic Patient Safety Report is created and distributed widely amongst management and leadership to articulate the creation of value.

Fostering Simulation Expertise

- **Enhance awareness**: Ensure prospective faculty members are aware of the simulation center. In addition to the existence of the simulation center it is also important to articulate the support it provides to faculty members. Consider inviting perspective simulation based teachers to a tour, or perhaps to attend or participate in successful simulation programs to stimulate further interest.
- **Develop a comprehensive faculty training program**: Provide educators and prospective simulation faculty members with the necessary skills and knowledge to confidently utilize simulation. This could involve workshops, online modules, or mentorship opportunities with experienced simulation facilitators.
- **Address specific needs and concerns**: Through surveys or focus groups, identify the specific challenges and learning preferences of potential simulation educators. Tailor the training program to address these needs and ensure it fosters confidence and a positive attitude towards simulation-based learning.

Overcoming Barriers

- **Technological challenges**: Identify and address potential technological barriers, such as equipment limitations or software issues. Collaborate with the IT department or simulation specialist team to ensure smooth operation and reliable support for simulation technology. Try to limit the amount of technical expertise that the faculty needs to provide by supporting them with such services when possible.
- **Psychological challenge**: Acknowledge the additional workload that implementing simulation might initially create. Offer practical solutions like scheduling dedicated time for training and development. Encourage faculty through a structured development process of courses and scenarios. Lead them to understand that an upfront investment in the creation ensure a smoother and less time consuming commitment when actually conducting the programs that are developed.

Structured Guidance for Simulation Educators

- **Define educator roles**: Clearly define the roles and responsibilities of simulation educators. This ensures a structured approach to training and provides clarity for both educators and participants.

- **Instructor guides**: Develop detailed instructor guides that provide clear instructions, learning objectives, and scenarios for simulation sessions. These guides serve as a valuable resource for both experienced and novice educators.

Peer-to-Peer Learning and Mentorship

- **Journal club for best practices**: Facilitate a journal club dedicated to simulation-based learning. This allows educators to stay updated on the latest research, share best practices, and explore innovative teaching methods.
- **Develop a peer learning network**: Establish a network within your organization where experienced simulation facilitators can share best practices and mentor colleagues who are new to simulation. This fosters a sense of community and facilitates knowledge transfer in a supportive environment.
- **Formal net-working sessions**: Provide regular opportunities for educators to share best practices, troubleshoot challenges, and learn from each other's experiences. Consider establishing a dedicated team or community of practice focused on simulation.

Enhancing Motivation and Engagement

- **Highlight the personal and professional benefits**: Emphasize how simulation skills can enhance not only patient care but also the personal and professional development of educators. Share examples of how simulation has helped colleagues feel more confident and effective in their roles. This might be done by fostering them to present their work at national or international meetings.
- **Recognize and celebrate achievements**: Acknowledge and celebrate the successful implementation of simulation programs and the contributions of actively involved educators. This fosters a sense of accomplishment and motivates continued participation.
- **Assist faculty with data collection**: Develop a system that allows faculty to track their teaching activities as well as the feedback they received from students. This serves as an excellent resource to allow them to report their simulation efforts to their superiors as needed for documentation of their efforts, as well as supporting evidence for an academic career promotion support.

By implementing these strategies, you can create a collaborative and supportive environment that encourages the active participation of your colleagues in healthcare simulation. Remember, successful implementation requires not only acquiring equipment and technology but also fostering a culture of innovation and continuous learning among your fellow healthcare professionals. Working together, you can leverage the power of simulation to create a positive impact on patient care, staff development, and the overall success of your organization.

Reference

WISER News and Updates. *WISER*. Accessed February 23, 2024. https://www.wisersimulation.org/news/

Chapter 14
Online Resources for Simulation Educators

Abstract This chapter explores a comprehensive collection of resources tailored for simulation educators, offering a valuable guide for professional development and scenario enrichment. The chapter provides an extensive list of online links, courses, and repositories specifically curated to enhance the knowledge and skills of simulation educators. These resources cover diverse topics, including scenario design, debriefing techniques, technology integration, and educational best practices. Emphasizing accessibility and relevance, the chapter aims to empower simulation educators to expand their expertise and stay abreast of the latest advancements in the field. Whether a novice or an experienced educator, this compilation serves as a go-to reference, fostering continuous learning and elevating the quality of simulation-based education. Access the provided link to embark on a journey of ongoing education and resource discovery tailored to simulation educators' needs and aspirations.

Keywords Online resources · Simulation educators · Professional development

This chapter explores a collection of resources tailored for simulation educators, offering a valuable professional and scenario development guide. The chapter provides an extensive list of online links and repositories specifically curated to enhance the knowledge and skills of simulation educators. The chapter aims to empower simulation educators to expand their expertise and stay updated on the latest advancements in the field.

14.1 The Society for Simulation in Healthcare

Established in 2004, the Society for Simulation in Healthcare (SSH) is a leading professional organization dedicated to promoting the use of simulation in healthcare education, assessment, and research (https://www.ssih.org/).

T. Tangpaisarn et al., *Navigating Healthcare Simulation*,
SpringerBriefs in Education, https://doi.org/10.1007/978-3-031-81265-1_14

Purpose: The SSH is driven by a core mission: to improve patient care by fostering the development and implementation of high-quality simulation programs across the healthcare spectrum by:

- **Promoting best practices**: The SSH advocates for using evidence-based practices and methodologies in simulation-based learning.
- **Advocacy and awareness**: The organization promotes the benefits of simulation to healthcare institutions, policymakers, and the public.
- **Facilitating collaboration**: The SSH fosters a community for healthcare professionals involved in simulation, encouraging knowledge sharing and collaboration.
- **Supporting research**: The SSH actively supports research efforts to advance the healthcare simulation field.

Content: The SSH website offers a comprehensive collection of resources for its members and the broader healthcare community:

- **Professional Development**: Educational programs, workshops, and webinars provide opportunities for members to enhance their skills and knowledge in simulation design, facilitation, and debriefing.
- **Research Information**: The SSH provides resources and support for conducting research related to simulation in healthcare. This includes access to research grants and opportunities to publish findings.
- **Credentialing**: The SSH offers opportunities to earn certifications in healthcare simulation, such as the Certified Healthcare Simulation Educator (CHSE) and the Certified Healthcare Simulation Operations Specialist (CHSOS).
- **Accreditation**: Recognizing the importance of quality standards, the SSH offers an accreditation program for healthcare simulation programs that meet established criteria.
- **Publications**: Members gain access to **Simulation in Healthcare** journal, featuring research articles, case studies, and best practice recommendations.

Target Audience: The SSH caters to a diverse range of professionals within the healthcare simulation field:

- **Healthcare educators**: Simulation specialists, faculty members, instructors, and program directors responsible for designing, delivering, and evaluating simulation-based learning experiences.
- **Healthcare professionals**: Physicians, nurses, allied health professionals, and other practitioners who utilize simulation for training and skill development.
- **Simulation operations professionals**: These individuals are dedicated to the support of simulation educational programs and the smooth operations of simulation facilities and the management of technology and equipment.
- **Researchers**: Individuals conducting research to evaluate the effectiveness of simulation in healthcare education and to advance the field as a whole.

By offering a wealth of resources, facilitating professional development, and promoting collaboration, the SSH empowers its members and the broader healthcare community to leverage simulation as a powerful tool for improving patient care.

14.2   International Nursing Association for Clinical Simulation and Learning (INACSL)

The International Nursing Association for Clinical Simulation and Learning (INACSL) is crucial in advancing healthcare simulation. One of their key initiatives is developing and promoting the Healthcare Simulation Standards of Best Practice™. Their focus is primarily on undergraduate and graduate nursing school education simulation (https://www.inacsl.org/healthcare-simulation-standards).

Purpose: The INACSL's Healthcare Simulation Standards of Best Practice (HSSOBP™) was created with a multi-faceted purpose:

- **Standardization**: These standards establish a set of best practices that function as benchmarks for evaluating the quality of simulation practices within healthcare education.
- **Evidence-Based Practices**: The standards are grounded in research and provide a framework for implementing simulation programs with a strong foundation in evidence-based practices.
- **Recognition**: The INACSL offers a Healthcare Simulation Standards Endorsement program. This program recognizes healthcare institutions and organizations that excel in applying the HSSOBP™ within their simulation education programs.

Content: The INACSL's Healthcare Simulation Standards of Best Practice outlines four core components that are fundamental to effective and high-quality healthcare simulation:

- **Prebriefing (Preparation and Briefing)**: This standard emphasizes the importance of thorough preparation and clear communication before a simulation event.
- **Facilitation**: This aspect focuses on the facilitator's role in effectively guiding learners through the simulation experience.
- **Debriefing**: Effective debriefing is a cornerstone of simulation-based learning. This standard emphasizes creating a safe and supportive environment for reflection and analysis after a simulation event.
- **Professional Integrity**: This core principle highlights the importance of ethical conduct, qualified personnel, and ongoing professional development within healthcare simulation programs.

Target Audience: The INACSL's HSSOBP™ cater to a broad audience within the healthcare simulation field:

- **Healthcare educators**: This includes simulation educators, faculty, and instructors responsible for designing and delivering simulation training programs.
- **Healthcare institutions and organizations**: Hospitals, medical schools, and other healthcare entities that utilize simulation-based learning in their educational programs.

By establishing these comprehensive standards, INACSL provides a valuable roadmap for educators, institutions, and all stakeholders involved in healthcare simulation. The Healthcare Simulation Standards of Best Practice contribute to a more standardized and evidence-based approach to simulation education, ultimately leading to improved patient outcomes.

14.3   HealthySimulation.com

HealthySimulation.com is a comprehensive resource hub for anyone interested in the ever-evolving world of healthcare education (https://www.healthysimulation.com).

Purpose: HealthySimulation.com was established with a mission to be the leading online resource for healthcare simulation by:

- **Centralizing information**: Providing a one-stop shop for news, updates, and educational materials related to healthcare simulation.
- **Facilitating knowledge sharing**: Creating a platform for educators, practitioners, and learners to connect, share best practices, and stay informed about the latest advancements in simulation-based learning.
- **Supporting professional development**: Offering a wide range of resources to help individuals enhance their skills and knowledge in healthcare simulation.

Content: HealthySimulation.com boasts a rich collection of content catering to various aspects of healthcare simulation:

- **News & Updates**: The website features daily updates on the latest developments, trends, and research findings in the field.
- **Continuing Education**: Educators and learners can access online courses, webinars, and other resources for professional development in simulation-based education.
- **Job Listings**: The website facilitates career exploration by providing a platform for healthcare simulation professionals to discover job opportunities.
- **Research Highlights**: Summaries of recent research studies keep users informed about the evolving evidence base supporting simulation-based learning.
- **Conference Recaps**: Users can stay up to date on past and upcoming conferences related to healthcare simulation.
- **Product Demos**: Explore the latest simulation products and technologies showcased on the website.

- **Vendor Listings**: Access a directory of companies involved in developing and supplying simulation equipment and resources.
- **Free Resources**: A treasure trove of downloadable content caters to diverse learning needs, including simulation scenarios for various healthcare disciplines (e.g., nursing, surgery), patient simulation tools and games to enhance training experiences, and debriefing guides to facilitate reflection and analysis after simulation activities

Target Audience: HealthySimulation.com caters to a broad audience within the healthcare simulation ecosystem:

- **Healthcare educators**: Simulation specialists, faculty members, and instructors responsible for designing, implementing, and evaluating simulation programs.
- **Healthcare professionals**: Nurses, physicians, and other practitioners can utilize the website to enhance their skills and knowledge through simulation-based learning resources.
- **Students and trainees**: Medical, nursing, and allied health students can explore simulation scenarios and resources relevant to their fields of study.
- **Industry professionals**: Individuals involved in developing and supplying simulation technologies and equipment can leverage the website for marketing and networking.

By offering a diverse range of content and fostering a collaborative environment, HealthySimulation.com empowers individuals across the spectrum of healthcare simulation. Whether you're a seasoned educator, a curious student, or a professional in the simulation industry, this website is a valuable resource to support your learning, development, and connection to the ever-growing field of healthcare simulation.

14.4 Simulating Healthcare

Simulating Healthcare, a blog dedicated to simulation, is a valuable platform for educators, practitioners, and anyone interested in the field to delve deeper into healthcare simulation (https://simulatinghealthcare.net/).

Purpose: Simulating Healthcare was established with a mission to foster a vibrant community around healthcare simulation by:

- **Disseminating knowledge**: Sharing insights, best practices, and recent developments in healthcare simulation through informative blog posts.
- **Promoting discussion**: Encouraging dialogue and exchange of ideas among simulation educators and learners through comments and forum discussions.
- **Enhancing practice**: Providing practical guidance and strategies to help educators design and implement effective simulation programs.

Content: Simulating Healthcare offers a diverse range of content to cater to the evolving needs of its audience:

- **Blog posts**: The core of the blog lies in its informative and insightful articles. These posts explore various themes related to simulation-based learning in healthcare, including:

  - Design and implementation of simulation programs
  - Debriefing techniques for effective post-simulation analysis
  - Utilizing simulation for specific healthcare disciplines (e.g., nursing, medicine)
  - The role and importance of simulation technicians in facilitating realistic scenarios
  - Ethical considerations in simulation-based education

- **Resources**: Beyond blog posts, the website provides additional resources to support learning and development in simulation education:

  - Links to relevant articles and research publications
  - Presentations and downloadable materials

- **Categories**: Easy navigation is facilitated by categorizing content based on specific focus areas within healthcare simulation.

Target Audience: Simulating Healthcare caters to a broad audience with a shared interest in healthcare simulation:

- **Healthcare educators**: Simulation specialists, faculty members, and instructors responsible for designing and delivering simulation training programs across various healthcare disciplines.
- **Healthcare practitioners**: Nurses, physicians, and other healthcare professionals who utilize simulation-based learning to enhance their clinical skills and decision-making abilities.
- **Students and trainees**: Individuals enrolled in healthcare programs or rotations incorporating simulation as a learning tool.
- **General enthusiasts**: Anyone interested in learning more about the growing field of healthcare simulation and its impact on improving patient care.

Simulating Healthcare empowers stakeholders across the spectrum of healthcare simulation by providing a platform for knowledge sharing, discussion, and exploration. Whether you're a seasoned educator, a curious student, or someone seeking to understand the role of simulation in healthcare, this blog offers valuable insights and resources to support your journey.

14.5   EM Sim Cases

EM Sim Cases is a free online resource specifically designed for emergency medicine (EM) simulation education. Launched in 2015, it has fostered a collaborative environment for educators and learners worldwide (https://emsimcases.com/).

Purpose: EM Sim Cases was established to provide a centralized repository of high-quality, peer-reviewed simulation cases for emergency medicine professionals. This centralized approach aims to:

- **Reduce redundancy**: By offering a vast pool of cases, educators can leverage existing resources instead of recreating them from scratch.
- **Enhance accessibility**: Educators and learners worldwide gain free access to valuable simulation materials.
- **Promote collaboration**: The platform fosters a culture of knowledge sharing and collaboration within the EM simulation community.

Content: EM Sim Cases offers a rich collection of resources to support simulation-based learning in emergency medicine:

- **Peer-reviewed simulation cases**: The website's core lies in its extensive library of downloadable simulation cases. These cases cover various emergency scenarios, catering to diverse learning needs.
- **Educational articles**: Articles delve into various aspects of simulation-based education, providing educators with practical strategies and best practices.
- **Modifiable simulation template**: A user-friendly template assists educators in developing customized simulation cases.
- **Community forum**: The platform facilitates discussions and knowledge exchange among EM simulation educators.

Target Audience: EM Sim Cases caters to a broad audience within the emergency medicine simulation community:

- **Emergency medicine educators**: Instructors, simulation specialists, and faculty responsible for designing and delivering simulation training programs in emergency medicine settings.
- **Healthcare professionals**: Residents, fellows, and practicing physicians seeking to enhance their clinical skills and decision-making through simulation experiences.
- **Medical students**: Students enrolled in emergency medicine rotations or programs can utilize case scenarios to prepare for future clinical encounters.

By providing a comprehensive range of resources and fostering a collaborative environment, EM Sim Cases empower educators to design effective simulation programs and equip learners with valuable skills for emergency situations.

14.6   The University of Washington's Simulation Team Training Toolkit

The University of Washington's Interprofessional Education Collaborative (IPEC) recognizes the crucial role of teamwork in healthcare. Their Simulation Team Training Toolkit addresses this need by providing educators with resources to develop and implement effective interprofessional simulation (IPS) training programs (https://collaborate.uw.edu/online-training-and-resources/simulation-team-training-toolkit/).

Purpose: The Simulation Team Training Toolkit was created to equip healthcare educators with the knowledge and tools necessary to design and deliver impactful IPS programs by:

- **Promoting interprofessional collaboration**: The toolkit emphasizes the importance of fostering teamwork and communication skills among healthcare professionals from diverse disciplines.
- **Enhancing patient care**: IPS training aims to improve collaboration and contribute to better patient outcomes through coordinated care.
- **Providing a practical framework**: The toolkit offers educators a step-by-step approach to developing and implementing IPS programs within their institutions.

Content: The Simulation Team Training Toolkit provides a comprehensive resource package for educators:

- **Overview of IPS**: The toolkit lays the foundation by explaining the concept of interprofessional simulation and its benefits in healthcare education.
- **Framework for Development and Implementation**: This section serves as a roadmap, guiding educators through designing, implementing, and evaluating IPS programs.
- **Resources:**
  - Case studies: Educators can leverage pre-developed case studies or use the toolkit's guidance to create scenarios tailored to specific learning objectives.
  - Debriefing tools: Effective debriefing is a critical element of simulation learning. The toolkit offers resources to facilitate constructive discussions and analysis after simulation experiences.
  - Evaluation materials: The toolkit provides guidance and tools to assess the effectiveness of the IPS training program.
- **TeamSTEPPS® Framework**: The toolkit highlights the **TeamSTEPPS®** framework, a widely used approach that provides a common language and structure for effective teamwork in healthcare settings.

Target Audience: The Simulation Team Training Toolkit primarily targets healthcare educators involved in developing and delivering interprofessional simulation-based training programs:

- **Simulation educators**: Individuals who design and facilitate simulation experiences for interprofessional healthcare professionals.
- **Faculty members**: Instructors responsible for incorporating simulation into interprofessional education curriculums across various disciplines.
- **Program directors**: Leaders overseeing healthcare education programs who seek to integrate interprofessional simulation as a valuable learning tool.

The toolkit is a valuable resource for educators seeking to understand and implement interprofessional simulation training. It offers a foundational framework and practical tools to cultivate effective collaboration among future healthcare teams.

14.7 Summary

This chapter has provided a brief overview of a sampling of valuable online resources available to healthcare simulation educators. While these resources offer a great starting point, many additional resources, information, and tools are available to support you in your role.

References

EM Sim Cases. Published December 15, 2023. Accessed March 12, 2024. https://emsimcases.com/
Healthcare Simulation | Medical Simulation | Nursing Simulation | HealthySimulation.com. Accessed March 12, 2024. https://www.healthysimulation.com
Healthcare Simulation Standards of Best Practice™. Accessed March 12, 2024. https://www.inacsl.org/healthcare-simulation-standards
Simulating Healthcare. A blog dedicated to discussions and relevant things regarding simulation in healthcare in healthcare. Accessed March 12, 2024. https://simulatinghealthcare.net/
Simulation Team Training Toolkit | Collaborate. Accessed March 12, 2024. https://collaborate.uw.edu/online-training-and-resources/simulation-team-training-toolkit/
Society for Simulation in Healthcare. Accessed March 12, 2024. https://www.ssih.org/

Chapter 15
The WISER Way

Abstract This chapter delves into the success story of the WISER, spotlighting the Simulation Center in Pittsburgh renowned for its innovative approach and transformative impact on healthcare education. The chapter provides an in-depth exploration of the center's origins, mission, and core principles that have propelled it to prominence in the field of simulation-based training. From state-of-the-art facilities to cutting-edge methodologies, the narrative unfolds the key elements contributing to WISER's success. Drawing on real-world experiences and lessons learned, this chapter serves as a blueprint for simulation centers aspiring to emulate the achievements of WISER. Whether a simulation enthusiast or a healthcare education professional, this insightful account offers inspiration and practical insights into the distinctive journey of WISER. Discover the unique identity, accomplishments, and the driving philosophy behind the success of this distinguished simulation center in Pittsburgh.

Keywords WISER · Simulation Center · Pittsburgh

The Winter Institute for Simulation, Education, and Research, also known as WISER, is a healthcare simulation training and research facility that is a partnership of the University of Pittsburgh Schools of Health Sciences and the UPMC Health System. WISER's mission is WISER is dedicated to the advancement of healthcare simulation and education to improve patient safety, education, mentorship, systems design, and research to enhance the high-quality delivery of healthcare.

© The Author(s), under exclusive license to Springer Nature Switzerland AG 2025   113
T. Tangpaisarn et al., *Navigating Healthcare Simulation*,
SpringerBriefs in Education, https://doi.org/10.1007/978-3-031-81265-1_15

15.1 WISER History

In the early 1990s, Dr. Peter Winter, the chairman of the Department of Anesthe-siology and Critical Care Medicine at the University of Pittsburgh, recognized the importance of establishing a simulation center to train department personnel. The department obtained a simulator for over $250,000, which was essentially the only commercial simulator available at the time. They also acquired computers and addi-tional equipment. In 1994, the simulation center was launched on the third floor of Montefiore University Hospital (https://www.wisersimulation.org/; https://www.upmc.com/about/why-upmc/quality/patient-safety/wiser).

The simulation center had arrangements to simulate an operating room, an ICU bed, or a bay in the emergency department. To complete the picture, anesthesia machines, monitors, and ventilators were also obtained. Over the next four years, a team of faculty members developed a broad range of curricula, which included performance evaluations using various components such as the internet, CD-ROM, Palm-based, and digital video-based.

In 1996, Drs. Rene Gonzales and John Schaefer designed and patented a difficult-airway simulator that was more functional, affordable, and portable than the existing commercial version. A Texas-based company, Medical Plastics Laboratory, which was later acquired by the Laerdal Corporation, manufactured this new simulator (AirMan) commercially. The core functionality of their work was incorporated into a cost effective full-scale human simulator (SimMan) which was commercially launched in 2000.

15.2 WISER Objectives

By incorporating simulation-based training and other state-of-the-art educational techniques, WISER seeks to create a safer environment for patients by providing healthcare professionals and students with opportunities to practice and enhance their skills in a controlled, risk-free environment. This approach allows them to develop and refine their competencies without compromising patient well-being.

In addition to prioritizing patient safety, WISER also explores ways to enhance the efficiency of healthcare delivery by evaluating and implementing innovative educa-tional and assessment methods. Through rigorous research and practical application, WISER serves as a laboratory for investigating the effectiveness of simulation-based training and other instructional approaches, aiming to identify and disseminate best practices for healthcare education.

Furthermore, WISER recognizes the importance of creating comprehensive education programs that cater to the diverse needs of healthcare providers at various stages of their careers, from students to practicing professionals. By developing simulation-based training programs and other educational initiatives, WISER aims to foster the development of competencies across multiple domains, ensuring that healthcare providers are equipped with the knowledge, skills, and attitudes necessary to provide high-quality care.

Lastly, WISER plays a crucial role in nurturing and mentoring future generations of healthcare educators and researchers passionate about creating, improving, and evaluating simulation-based teaching programs. By providing a supportive and collaborative environment, WISER contributes to the growth and development of these individuals, empowering them to drive innovation and advance the field of healthcare education.

15.3 WISER Clinical Simulation Courses

WISER offers a variety of simulation education courses that can be browsed based on participant type, CME courses, or department. The departments include anesthesiology, cardiology, cardiothoracic surgery, children's hospital, critical care medicine, biological sciences, advanced practice providers, pharmacy, internal medicine, pulmonary, allergy and critical care medicine, emergency medicine, graduate nursing, undergraduate nursing, nursing CME, obstetrics, gynecology and reproductive services, pediatrics, rehabilitation, psychology, radiology, dental medicine, and surgery. Each department offers several medical simulation courses to enhance knowledge and understanding in the related field.

WISER also provides faculty and staff development courses for simulation educators and administrators, designed to help them improve their simulation training skills. These courses include Improving Simulation Instructional Methods (iSIM), Facilitator Training Series: Introduction to Debriefing, and Healthcare Simulation Operations Specialist Training Program (TechSim) and many other programs. The iSIM fundamentals program is a two-day internationally recognized course created by WISER at the University of Pittsburgh and the Gordon Center for Research in Medical Education at the University of Miami. The course focuses on teaching fundamental skills and abilities for delivering simulation-based healthcare education using various techniques and technologies. The program emphasizes hands-on activities and active participation to maximize skill acquisition. The primary audience for this course is healthcare educators who want to enhance their skills as instructors in simulation education. The class group size is kept small for maximum participation.

The Facilitator Training Series: Introduction to Debriefing course is designed to introduce facilitators to various facilitation and debriefing techniques. Participants learn the skills required to become more effective facilitators through a mixture of didactics and hands-on activities.

Finally, the Healthcare Simulation Operations Specialist Training Program (TechSim) is designed to educate healthcare simulation operations specialists on the key tasks associated with the daily operations and maintenance of a simulation center.

15.4   WISER Visiting Scholars Programs

Two WISER visiting scholars programs are available: the fellowship program and the preceptorship program. The fellowship program is a comprehensive one to two-year curriculum incorporating electives, workshops, course observations, the WISER Foundation, and a scholarly project. The program is tailored to those interested in a broad range of topics, such as simulation center operations, information technology, administration, and curriculum development. Participants in the fellowship program will receive personalized support from subject matter experts who will assist with project completion and provide guidance on research, curriculum development, or a combination of topics. Participants will also have the opportunity to integrate into WISER's network of simulation education expertise.

The preceptorship program is a structured curriculum designed for individuals interested in a one to eleven-month curriculum that includes electives, workshops, course observations, and the WISER Foundation. Like the fellowship program, it covers a wide range of topics, such as simulation center operations, information technology, administration, and curriculum development. The program is facilitated by subject matter experts who will provide participants with the guidance required to complete the program successfully.

References

Winter Institute for Simulation, Education, and Research. WISER. Accessed September 26, 2024. https://www.wisersimulation.org/

WISER | UPMC Quality, Safety & Innovation. UPMC | Life Changing Medicine. Accessed September 26, 2024. https://www.upmc.com/about/why-upmc/quality/patient-safety/wiser